I AM ENOUGH- INTO THE SHADOWS

HEALING A BROKEN BODY VOLUME 2

BY

MICHAEL PESTANO

NOTE TO THE READER

Disclaimer: *This book is not intended as a substitute for psychological services or implied to be a substitute for professional medical advice, diagnosis, or treatment of any kind. Readers should consult with a physician or other health care professional before beginning or making any life changes. The author expressly disclaims responsibility for any liability, loss, or risk—personal or otherwise—which is incurred, directly or indirectly, as a consequence of the use and application of any of the contents of this book. No specific claims or guarantees are being made as to the outcome or results incurred from applying ideas and recommendations set forth in this book. Results vary as do individuals. In other words, as a person who is responsible for your own life, you must be responsible in reading this book. No one is responsible for you but yourself. By reading this book you acknowledge you are ready and willing to own full responsibility for your life and decisions.*

Book cover photo by Jhenny Morales Evans

DEDICATION

I believe in the spirit of universal love and positivity. I believe in angels, ascended masters and my own spiritual guides. I believe in the greatness within humanity in each and every one of us. There is a beauty and power that lies within me that I have discovered and haven't fully tapped into and it is in everywhere and in everything. And to those who I call angels in my life that I have experienced unconditional love, kindness, compassion, friendship, and positivity I thank you. The world needs more of these beautiful beings of love and light. instead of fear, polarization, superstition, doubt, psychological and emotional negativity. My hope is to bring this book to those who have never felt yet that they are not capable of healing a broken body from within. But know that you are capable of healing through the intention of your spirit with hope, faith, and courage.

To my parents, Jaime and Theresa Pestano, my siblings Gabriel, Maritess, and Mia. You all have been my bedrock of love, faith, support, and teachers in my life. My dearest sister Maritess, thank you for creating those special goodies that helped me heal and recover.

To my coach, teacher and best friend Radhaa Nilia. You came into my life when I needed support the most. Your unconditional love, friendship, kindness, long distance coaching and healing, compassion, and wisdom gave me the strongest foundation to heal and transform.

To my Lemurian Code Healing guide, coach and shaman healer Maya The Shaman, your knowledge and wisdom in regards to the practical healing tools you have provided such as a plant-based lifestyle and herbal healing protocol allowed my body to heal internally. The massive damage inflicted was cleared miraculously.

To my dear soul sister, Akashic Records guide, and healer Teza Zialcita. Your guidance, love, wisdom, and support while I was healing in Vancouver is much appreciated.

And to all of you who I consider my spiritual brother and sisters around the world with whom I resonated with and learned, worked, spread love, and experienced joy and happiness, let's all continue to inspire the world together.

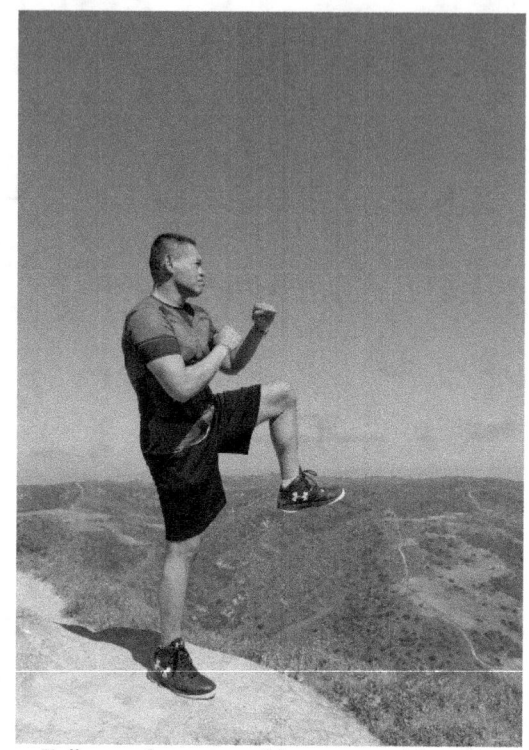

Follow and connect with me on social media:

Facebook – facebook.com/lightwarrior88

Instagram- @iamenough888

Twitter- @OurEvolution888

LinkedIn – Mike Pestano

TABLE OF CONTENTS

ACKNOWLEDGMENTS

To those amazing people who have contributed and are instrumental in the making of my book I'd like to provide credit to whom this is due.

To my dearest friend and business mentor Emma Tiebens, you encouraged me to write about my story back in 2014 and guided and inspired me to pursue my dreams.

To my dear friends Nicole Parker, Raziel Arcega, Teza Zialcita, Jake and Christian Rosario, Arleen Arce Tan, Tracy and Derek Tangedal, Gigi Grey-Ricarse, Crisanta Sampang, and the Big Shift crew,

Rey and Cely Fortaleza of Reyfort Media Group, and my dear cousin Patrick Dinglasan. Thank you!

To my business associates Sarah Staniforth, Rafic Sidani, and the rest of the Ecoideas Canada team thank you for your love, friendship and support while I was a part of the Western Canada team. A special recognition to Donna Vachon for introducing me to this company.

You all inspired me to create this second book and share it to the world. Your love and support during difficult and challenging times is much appreciated.

Letters of Gratitude

"Do all the good you can. By all the means you can. In all the ways you can. In all the places you can. At all the times you can. To all the people you can. As long as ever you can." – John Wesley

My dear friend Emma Tiebens, said it best; "Individually strong, together invincible." My journey into successful healing wouldn't have happened without the amazing people that came into my life. They have each given so much of themselves and have enriched my life and given joy, happiness, love, friendship and support. My sincerest gratitude and love to each one of you.

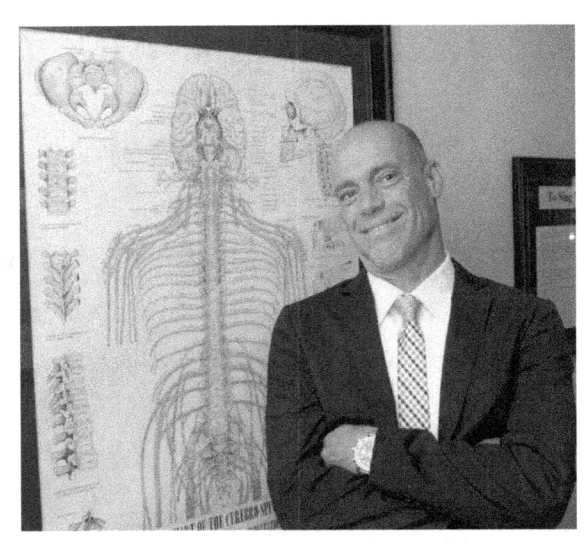

DR. BILLY DEMOSS

Dear Dr. Billy,

My journey to health began with you in early 2011 and your impact has been life-transforming. Your passion for life, living your truth, commitment to serving your patients, and tireless advocacy for a healthy and happy lifestyle rubbed off on me deeply. You were not just my chiropractor whom I saw for weekly adjustments. Your expertise in chiropractic was invaluable in setting me up for success with my health.

Those regular health seminars you and your fellow health care practitioners held at your office enriched my knowledge on health and nutrition. Those seminars gave me a great foundation and helped me with designing personal healing protocols that to this day keeps me healthy and happy. Beyond that your greatest impact in my life lies in inspiring me to start living my truth with passion. I saw your daily posts on social media and you backed your talk with your actions and results. Thank you to you and Maryjane for always inviting me to your California Jam chiropractic conventions. They opened my eyes and heart to my own mission and purpose. We are all here for a short time on earth and it's important to live it as if it's your last.

I've met many people and you're one of the very few who was truly authentic and transparent. That's a rare trait to have in a world that would rather have us be just like everyone else. Thank you for your friendship and inspiring me to be the change I want to be. Carpe Diem!

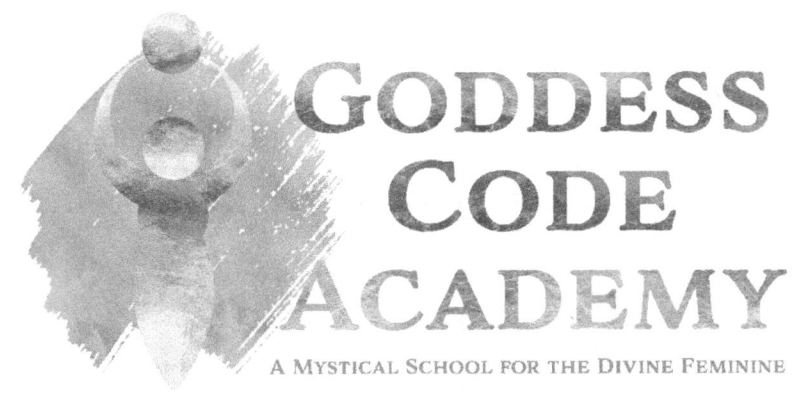

RADHAA NILIA OF GODDESS CODE

ACADEMY™

Dear Radhaa,

"Healing is a choice." Timeless words indeed from a dear friend, trusted mentor and coach that you are. Your light and love are a beacon to many who are lost in the darkness. You came into my life when

I needed support the most. Your unconditional love, friendship, kindness, long distance coaching and healing, compassion, and wisdom gave me the strongest foundation to heal and transform.

This book wouldn't have been possible without you. Your original Goddess Code Activations™ through Goddess Code Academy™ was the massive spark that propelled me into my transformation in 2012 and the foundation of my healing journey from 2013 to 2015.

You helped me clear negative beliefs, blockages and lineage wounds and awaken the feminine gifts and energies in me. These energies were activated in me and worked through me as a guide towards finding the physical resources I needed to heal and move forward. It balanced my overly dominant wounded masculinity and shifted it into a beautifully harmonious alignment with the Divine Feminine. This holistic education and empowerment also served to have me re-establish my deep connection with Mother Gaia and nature. You inspired me to further explore my talents of creativity, art, and love for writing. Most of all you helped me find my one true life path, higher purpose, and ultimately go enthusiastically for my dreams.

People come into our lives for a reason and I am grateful that you came into my life. Through this journey I came to understand that working in service of others and the greater good of humanity and the world brings abundance, blessings, true joy and happiness. The process of healing involves a commitment to doing the work internally with courage, persistence, passion, and purpose. I learned that the answers were inside of me and I shone the light in the shadows of my scarred and wounded self to heal it and let go of the fears that limited me. The hallmark of a mentor and coach is how a student applies the lessons learned to succeed and reach their goals. Thank you for your friendship, your light and your unconditional love. Namaste.

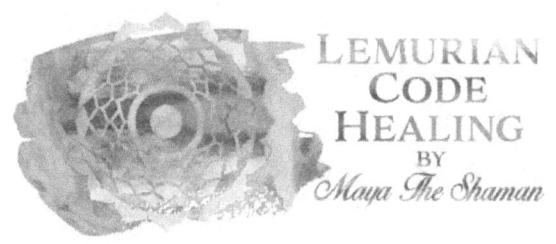

MAYA THE SHAMAN OF LEMURIAN CODE

HEALING

Dear Maya,

You have been there with me since 2012 as a healer and coach who helped me through my first transformation. Your deep knowledge and expertise of the ancient healing arts through your original Lemurian Code Healings™ modality, wisdom, intuition, love, compassion and generosity helped me purge lifetimes of the negative energies that were stuck inside of me and lead me to a clarity unparalleled. When I fell seriously ill in 2013 it was through your expertise in a plant-based lifestyle and ayurvedic herbs and holistic healing knowledge that formed the foundation of my future healing protocol.

Initially, I was fearful when my illness manifested but I learned to let go of the fear and forge through the pain. I learned techniques on visualization and meditation where I saw myself fully recovered, whole and complete. Thank you for helping to purge the internal conflicts and beliefs that no longer served me for my highest good.

The road to recovery spanned over three years and daily internal work that I would then apply to balance my external existence. Through this awakening and deep healing inside of me I became that warrior that transmuted the limitations and dysfunctions my old self had placed on me. I continue to evolve and do the work necessary to enrich society and make this world a better place. Thank you for everything you have taught me and activated in me. I happily continue this work with a grateful heart. Namaste.

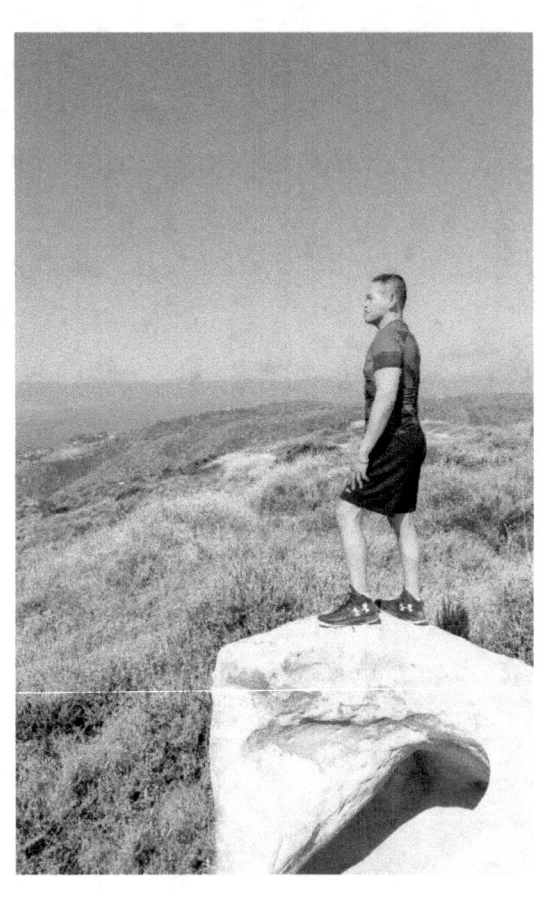

Introduction: Into The Shadows

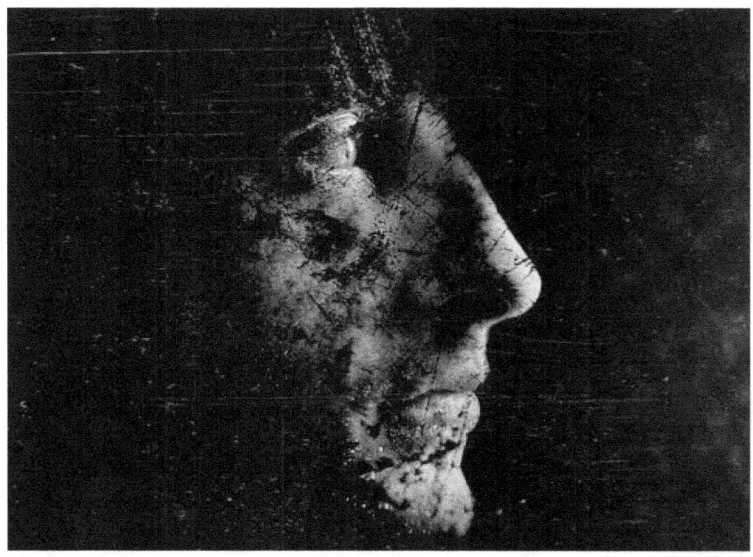

"Part of the healing process is sharing with people who care." - Jerry Cantrell

We are conditioned to fear the dark. We fear the unknown. We fear change and we are conditioned to stay in a comfort zone where nothing grows. Many of us would rather live through a life of pain without growth. But not me. I grew up in a culture, a society, and a family structure where risk was frowned upon. Yet in the hearts of all men and women exists a true self that became relegated to the shadows. Through this journey of transformation and evolution which began when I shed the weight and reversed the diabetes that threatened to keep me prisoner I learned that this adventure called life was just beginning.

The year 2012 was a year wherein I felt the best I had ever been in mind, body, and spirit. Strength, stamina, and endurance were at an optimum physical level. My mental acuity and focus was also dramatically different than the last decade. And on the spiritual level I discovered new aspects about myself that I enthusiastically embraced and was determined to grow. Through my healers Radhaa

Nilia of Goddess Code Academy™ and Maya The Shaman I learned to heal, expunge, balance, and bring in new positive energies as I continued to evolve further. That year was the best of times and the worst of times and it would save me later on.

Other aspects of my life had been going through tremendous upheaval and everything around me was crumbling down. My marriage had spiralled downwards mostly caused by lack of communication, financial and economic distress, and emotional disconnect. It would be easy to point fingers at each other but that never solves anything. Everyone has their flaws and shortcomings and I'm just as flawed as everyone else on this planet. When it's happening at the moment, both our emotions tend to get high-pitched and anger and jealousy would rear its head through the ego personality. I'm grateful I went through that spiritual and energetic healing process as that was the only thing keeping me afloat.

We were losing our houses, our cars, our investments had been cashed out, we had filed for bankruptcy, and our savings were almost gone even after the injury settlement I had received a couple of years before. I found my solace in the gym through exercise and through the meditations and spiritual exercises learned from Radhaa and Maya. I had a great new supporting cast of friends through the Filipino Chamber of Commerce of Orange County and I had gone back out into the world. Even though I was active on social media it wasn't my full, true, and authentic self that I showed. I was burnt out from years and years of overwork and stress of trying to maintain our standard of living and it was crashing down that year.

In my first book I AM Enough- Healing A Broken Body, I detailed the journey I went through to lose the weight and reverse the type 2 diabetes that was wrecking me internally. The aftermath of that transformation was probably the happiest time of my life at that point. My body and mind had been resuscitated and revived with a strength and vigor I hadn't felt since I was in college. My spiritual evolution was just beginning and I could feel the tug of my soul calling for further transformation. I could hear and sense the whispers like a foreboding that I couldn't quite pinpoint yet. I was just enjoying and living the moment in a body and mind that felt two decades younger.

The winds of change were coming though and in a few more months in 2012 I would hurtle into a whole new world. I would first have to travel back to a place where I would face old haunting memories and events. I would come face-to-face with my own darkness and that wounded part of me that needed to fully heal. I knew that my healers Radhaa and Maya could take me up to a certain point. It would be up to me to forge on and do the internal work necessary to carry me through it all. That is everyone's responsibility. We have this tendency to look for others to heal and fix us and that the external world can somehow be the answers to all that hurts us.

My last healing session with Radhaa was in the first week of June of 2012 during the full moon. I had learned about and embraced how energy truly permeates our lives whether it be from the lunar energies, our sun that keeps us and our planet alive, and our connection to the entire universe and everything in it and beyond. I learned to internalize and look within on a regular basis. That last healing session was akin to a graduation ceremony of sorts and I remember that conversation we had at the end. She asked me if I was ready to do the work. I didn't know fully what she meant by that but on an internal level somehow my soul knew. I firmly said yes with conviction and determination and I had no fear at the time.

I continued with my regular workouts and my nutrition program was being fine-tuned even further. During that time, I had a goal of joining a physique contest in the masters' division. It was a lifelong dream I had since I was twelve years old to someday go up on stage and be like Arnold Schwarzenegger. Heck, it would make me so happy to get on the cover of one of the muscle and fitness magazines. It was part of my escape too from an unhappy environment. I had healed a lot of past hurts and failures and now I was coming face to face with the deeper layers of a fragile psyche.

All my health markers were perfect and my doctor was very impressed with my transformation. I was emboldened that I felt better and more alive than I had ever been. I thought I had solved everything and I felt invincible. How many middle-aged men can feel like that? Majority of my peers were resigned to the fact that they were aging and that taking prescription drugs was just a daily part of life. Even when they had seen the transformation I had gone through the first words I'd hear from them would be; "I can't. It's too hard. I'm old. I wish I was like you. I don't have the discipline. I've got too many injuries. Only you can do that." Why is a scarcity and a negative mindset so ingrained in many? What can be done to change that? I wanted to inspire them that age was just a number and that it would boil down to a mindset of positivity.

We've all been programmed to fear the darkness and shun it in favor of the light. In this life, we live on this earth and we cannot escape the duality of night and day. As much as we try and avoid the shadows and the darkness it always comes. It's been going on here for billions of years as our planet revolves around the sun. It is part of the circle of life. I used to be so afraid of the dark. In my first book I was terrified of being left alone in the dark until I was thirteen years old. I can thank my childhood nanny for instilling that fear of things and creatures that supposedly come out at night.

I grew out of that and became fascinated with just how much life exists and happens in the dark of night and under the sea. There surely must be an explanation of how life can exist thousands of meters under the sea or in the deepest and darkest caves above and below. I became fascinated with how much activity goes on at night and in the dark while we sleep. This is a fascinating and beautiful world we live in and I learned to appreciate it even more. I learned at that time that in the darkness there is pain and there is also growth. I just had to be reminded time and again.

Why do we fear the dark? Why do we fear change? It's always a part of our lives yet we try to escape and avoid it at all costs even when it means more pain. I was listening to Gary Zukav's Seat of the

Soul audiobook and he said something about ninety percent of our personality or ego would resist change even as ten percent would fight for change. There is one true constant in life and in time. Everything changes around us and that ten percent will eventually go past that resistance of the ninety percent. I was reminded of that and it's so true as I began my transformation back in 2011. There was that big part of me that didn't want to change but my ten percent was so loud, incessant, persistent, and relentless that I went on to lose that 107 pounds and reverse the type 2 diabetes naturally. Furthermore, the spiritual, mental, and emotional healing became the foundation for my transformation and evolution.

With that said, the next logical effect would be further change and it would happen in less than a year. I knew in my heart and soul that the winds of change were blowing harder and it would take me on another ride. Little did I know this ride would take me to the deepest depths of my soul and face the mortality of my earthly life.

Not only would I have to walk into the pitch-black darkness I would have to find a way to go through it. I would have to explore the darkest, innermost, savagely wounded part of me and be my own healer, hero and savior. There would be no turning back and I would need to rely on myself and the lessons and knowledge I had learned by myself, from my mentors and teachers, and my best friend.

I share with you this journey not from a technical standpoint about human diseases and conditions. It's also not about medications and their applications and dosages. Nor is it about a trendy diet and a one size fits all approach. We've been conditioned to think and believe in one solution, one remedy, one approach, and one way of solving challenges and problems in life. Life's not like that at all and I share my journey as a complete holistic approach much like the way I did my first transformation.

The health information I give in this book is based solely on my own personal experience. It shouldn't be interpreted as medical advice or instruction. Nor should it be used as a basis for any diagnosis or treatment and as a substitute for professional medical advice. What I did here and share with you now is my own complete and personal holistic and spiritual protocol to save my life.

Life is all about making choices and we make those choices either with fear or with faith. Fears are illusions we put in place to limit ourselves from our greatness. Our bodies have an infinite capacity to heal and this would be fully tested in this saga.

You will learn about a mysterious disease with no known cure. That's what the doctors said but I refused to accept it. Come with me now into the shadows and journey with hope, faith, and courage.

"Wounds don't heal the way you want them to, they heal the way they need to. It takes time for wounds to fade into scars. It takes time for the process of healing to take place. Give yourself that time. Give yourself that grace. Be gentle with your wounds. Be gentle with your heart. You deserve to heal." - Dele Olanubi

CHAPTER I- Hello Darkness

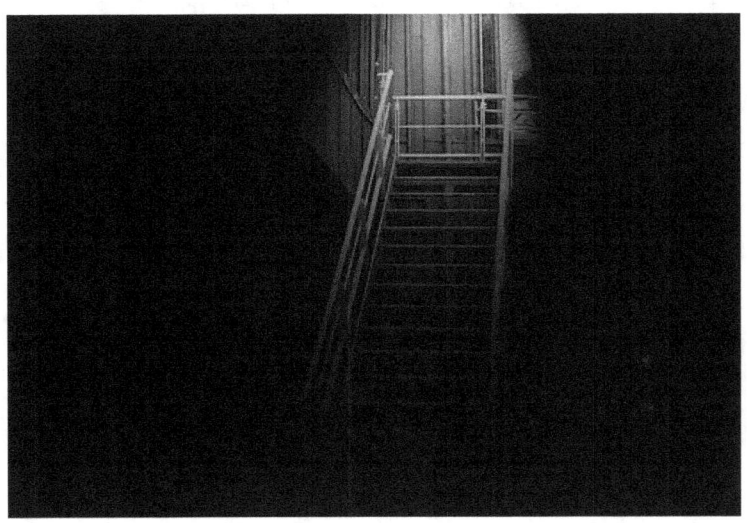

"In order for the light to shine so brightly, the darkness must be present." - Francis Bacon

This was definitely not what I had envisioned or even planned would happen to me. Finding myself lying in bed in a hospital in Anaheim, California. The weakness, deep intense pain, and exhaustion unlike anything I've ever felt. Hooked up with all kinds of tubes all over me and machines monitoring every aspect of life functions. Thoughts race through my mind replaying that darkness threatening to envelop my whole being and snuff out my lifeforce the first time it happened.

It's like descending deep into a cavern with fear gripping me and stripping me off the courage and numbing me. That night of April 29, 2013 would mark the beginning of a new journey unlike anything else. I had some early warning signs before it happened. I had just come back from a much-needed vacation in Vancouver, British Columbia in Canada. I had been away for a decade and I was happy to see my parents, my sisters, and old friends I had left behind. As I lay in that hospital bed in Anaheim Regional Hospital I was struggling to put all the pieces together what had caused my gallbladder and liver to be so acutely inflamed.

The initial diagnosis was chronic hepatitis along with a highly inflamed gallbladder. I had already been jaundiced for about 4 weeks prior to my hospitalization. Since my transformation the year before wherein I lost over 107 pounds and reversed type 2 diabetes I had been on an incredible high. Being in the best physical shape of my life was a happy and liberating time. My mind too was sharp unlike the previous years.

The first thing that came to my mind why my liver and gallbladder were damaged was maybe some kind of food poisoning. While I was in Vancouver I had indulged myself almost daily eating a lot of sushi and sashimi. Was it possible that the raw fish caused the inflammation? The blood tests for hepatitis A, B, and C were negative so there was a lot of unknown factors the doctors were trying to find out. They asked me to list all the nutritional supplements I had been taking which was extensive. One of the doctors thought it could be the supplements but he could not make a conclusion about it since I had been taking them for many years without adverse reactions. I had not been taking any drugs or steroids as he initially thought. One thing I never touched going all the way back to my high school and college years was drugs and steroids. He peppered me with questions about my alcohol intake. Yes, I drank beer, wine, and hard liquor when I was younger but mostly on social occasions. I wasn't the type to have beer and any other alcohol stored at home.

I was scheduled for more tests including a liver biopsy, MRI, and ultrasound of my abdomen. I was extremely weak and even with my high pain threshold the constant intensity of the pain assaulting me in my abdominal area was unbearable. The nurses and doctors offered to give me opioids but I refused. I knew that the inflammation in my liver and gallbladder was from something and I had to pinpoint where it all began. No more drugs! My thoughts flashed back to the time I had been taking a lot of powerful painkillers prescribed to me in 2010. I was taking Naproxen up to three times a day to ease the pain of the torn ligaments in my right elbow. I continued to take them up to the end of 2011 after surgery and rehabilitation. I should have asked more questions about the side effects of such powerful medications. Too late now to go back.

Then again, I had been taking over the counter pain relievers like Tylenol and Advil regularly since I was young. They were common drugs we popped whenever we had headaches, flu, muscle aches, sprains, and strains. In the Philippines there was this popular pain reliever analgesic called Alaxan that my mom always gave to us when we had any sign of pain symptoms. Lying in that hospital bed I was trying to piece together what could have caused my liver to be so highly inflamed. This was the most serious situation of my life and I was searching for answers. It was difficult to think between the pain and the extreme exhaustion plaguing me. I had put off going to the hospital for almost a month even after my doctor had diagnosed that I was already jaundiced.

I had signs that my body was starting to break down while I was in Vancouver and I chalked it up to the extreme stress I was under. My mom sensed something was amiss with me when she reached out in October of 2012. Call it a mother's instinct or intuition but she felt that energy. She called me and I finally broke down and told her what was going on with my life. I talked to my Dad too and I told them that I felt so lost and broken. My marriage was a disaster along with the rest of my personal life and financial situation. We were going to lose our home in Anaheim soon and six months prior to that we had already surrendered our investment property in Arizona. My retirement and stock plans had already been cashed out and my settlement from the elbow injury was running out. We had already filed for personal bankruptcy a couple of years before too and now we were going to lose everything.

I was down and almost out and what was keeping me going was the new knowledge I had learned from my healer friends Radhaa and Maya The

Shaman. Learning about meditation and going through powerful energy healing sessions with them helped save my life. There was so much more I learned from them that I would apply to my life that would transform me. In the meantime, I needed to get away from California as soon as possible. I would go back to Vancouver and reunite with my family and spend some time to heal. I stayed there for a couple of months and I felt rejuvenated. I came back to California looking forward to getting my life back on track. I had been offered a contract to be a business and social media consultant for a prominent natural pharmacy chain in Vancouver and I was set to go back until this happened. But there were signs and I ignored them thinking it wasn't anything serious. Those signs would manifest themselves soon in the form of jaundice and other internal complications.

As a typical guy not wanting to show any emotions and avoid showing signs of weakness I kept a facade up. I thought that I had worked on that particular aspect and my shadow-self came roaring back. On social media and to the outside world I had just transformed myself by losing over 107 pounds a year before and reversed my type 2 diabetes in the process. But there were signs and my social media posts showed glimpses of the discord that was simmering and smoldering. I knew I was peeling off layers and layers of emotions and feelings of discontent, anger, and frustration that had built up. This was what

Radhaa meant after my healing sessions months before that I would be peeling myself like an onion. Much like the waves of an ocean there would gentle ones and there would be stormy ones.

My dear friends Radhaa and Maya The Shaman were also imploring me in early April 2012 when I was diagnosed with jaundice to seek help from those who had healed it naturally. I didn't want to go to the hospital because I was afraid. The first reason was I did not have any health insurance and could not afford it. The second reason was I was afraid to find out what was really going on inside of me. Aside from being afraid my predilection for pride and stubbornness was rearing its head again. Deep down inside of me I was hoping that this was all just a nightmare and it would all go away. My ego was reasserting itself and now here I am lying in this bed scared and in extreme pain and exhaustion.

What were the symptoms that first began creeping in? The first immediate symptom I felt was extreme fatigue and it began during my trip to Vancouver. I continued my rigorous training at the Richmond Olympic Oval and I noticed it was getting harder to recover. I also noticed my pee getting darker and my stools were turning a greyish hue. I chalked it up to overtraining and that I was consuming a lot of raw fish from the sushi and sashimi. It would go on for a couple of days and then go back to normal after. But the fatigue was something else. I just felt so drained of energy for the most part of the day. I tried to sleep it off and I thought I was coming down with the flu but I had no fever. This would go on for the next several weeks and more ominous warning signs while I was on vacation for several days in Victoria.

My skin began to itch like crazy all over and I noticed it was scaly and getting so dry even with the copious amounts of moisturizing lotion and coconut oil I would slather. My eyes were turning a light yellow and my breasts began feeling really tender and tissue loose. I looked like I had gynecomastia also known as man-boobs. I would get chills out of the blue and would shiver uncontrollably during the night. I would be lying in bed in my sister's house in Richmond and I wouldn't have the strength to stand up for more than five seconds before plopping down on the bed. However, as mysteriously as these symptoms flared up they went away after several days.

The process would repeat itself when I got back to California in late March. We were in the midst of packing up all our belongings as we were losing our house to foreclosure and had to move out soon. It was a very stressful time for everyone in the house. What finally got me to go see a doctor on April 2, 2013 was the exhaustion was so debilitating I couldn't stand up for more than a few minutes. I somehow drove myself to see my doctor and when she saw me she looked shocked. I didn't realize I was already colored a yellowish-orange hue and in the natural lighting of her office she had me look at myself in the mirror. I looked like a pumpkin.

I still didn't want to go to the hospital since I had no insurance so she implored me to get a blood test done on the spot in her office. She wanted to see if it was a viral kind of hepatitis. I waited a couple of days and went back to her clinic to get the results. The lab results showed highly elevated liver enzymes and bilirubin. My AST was at 1880 u/l and my ALT was 3650 u/l and bilirubin of 7.8 mg/dl.

What this meant was that my liver and gallbladder were both compromised severely and bile was leaking into my bloodstream. She advised that this was beyond her expertise and I needed to go to the hospital. Thankfully the tests for Hepatitis A, B, and C were negative so I still refused. What was going on in my head was fear and lots of it. Everything that I had learned about going with the flow and being positive was now blocked and paralyzed with fear. Panic was setting in and I really felt at that time my whole world was really tumbling down to the lowest point. Here I am a few weeks away from losing our house and now I needed medical attention but I had no insurance. My American dream was becoming a full-fledged nightmare and all the nice and beautiful kumbaya feelings I had last year were replaced with this darkness enveloping me. Not just physically, but my mental and emotional state was shutting down to. Somehow, I was able to compose myself and told my doctor I'd heal it naturally. She reluctantly agreed to my request and gave me some printouts about jaundice. That would be the last time I'd see her and I went back home to tell my wife at that time what was going on.

I went home and told her and her mom and brother about my situation and they too were hesitant and afraid for me. I also shared with Radhaa and Maya what the results were and they referred me to someone they knew had healed jaundice naturally. Maya went further and recommended I use some ayurvedic herbs and remedies like ashwagandha, zeolite, triphala, and amalaki. I did research on the Internet about the types of foods and diets that may help. For the next three weeks I went on a fasting diet and only ate oatmeal with raw honey, egg whites, bananas, and lots of spinach and kale. My appetite wasn't like it was before so I'd be lucky to eat two meals at the maximum. I drank lots of water throughout the day and rested all throughout. I felt that I was making headway and my strength was improving.

On the night of April 29, 2013 I suddenly experienced severe pains in my upper abdomen that was more excruciating than anything I had ever felt before. It was much worse than the appendicitis I had in 1997 and it felt like there were thousands of hot needles trying to burst out of my stomach. My stool color too was ash grey and I said to myself this was really bad. I had my wife drive me to Anaheim Regional Memorial hospital that night and the admitting nurse had me taken in immediately.

Now here I am in the darkness of the hospital room with tubes and monitors connected all over me. Nurses would come in every hour to take my blood pressure and check my other vital signs. Every four hours another nurse would come in and draw blood from my right arm. I could hardly sleep with all that round-the-clock activity and to make it more harrowing I would hear the haunting sounds of screams of pain from people in other hospital rooms. It was all so surreal and I was calling out and asking silently to the universe and the angels if I had already descended into my own personal hell. I was calling out energetically to Radhaa and Maya The Shaman too because I was so afraid and alone. They were the ones I trusted the most and I remembered how a year before they had helped me through my transformational weight loss journey I shared in my first book.

I'd close my eyes and try to sleep as best as I could and the painkillers dripping slowly into my arm would alleviate the pain in my gut. Three days into my hospital stay the doctors had gone through so many tests already but no definitive answers. The positive aspect I took from all this was that my liver enzymes were more than fifty percent down from a month ago. It was definitely not Hepatitis A, B, or C but what was it?

One major hypothesis was that I may have a rare condition called Hemochromatosis and my doctor had me contact my parents in Vancouver to ask some questions. He hypothesized that the excess amount of iron found in my liver was from a genetic mutation. My body was absorbing too much iron from the food I was eating. When I went on my transformation program I consumed a lot of red meat and green leafy vegetables rich in iron. He wasn't able to narrow it down to that reason though.

He still clung on to his hypothesis that it may be hemochromatosis and that I may have in my DNA Northern European ancestry. It sounded quite far-fetched considering I was a Filipino with Spanish last name and I had predominantly Oriental features. I found out that I did have some British blood in me since my mom's great-grandmother was half-British. There were more tests that needed to be run though, and time was ticking fast and my condition was getting worse.

The other doctor was itching to have my gallbladder surgically removed but my liver was too highly inflamed and there was the risk of bleeding to death during surgery. It became a waiting game with my life on the line. Time to dig deeper than I have ever have before. Hello darkness my old friend. We meet again.

"Limitations live only in our minds. But if we use our imaginations, our possibilities become limitless." —Jamie Paolinetti

Chapter II –Life Is A Box Of Chocolates

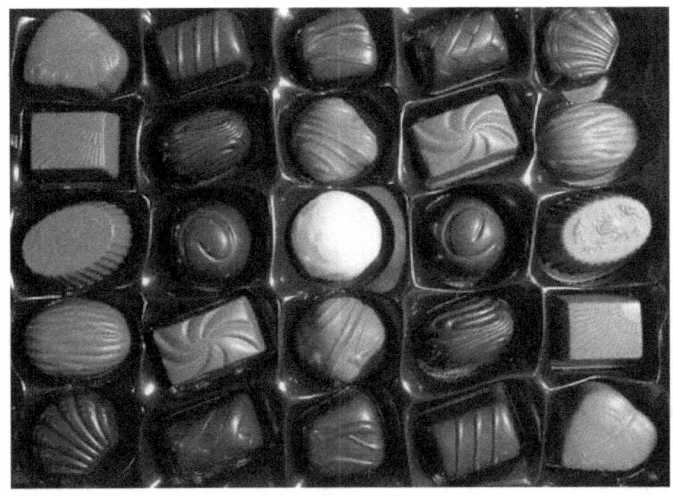

"Life is like a box of chocolates. You never know what you're gonna get." - Forrest Gump

That quote from my favorite movie Forrest Gump sums up my philosophy in life ever since I watched it. When you're actually living through the surprises in life that comes your way you ask yourself, "Why is this happening?" It sure as heck wasn't fun lying in bed in a hospital with tubes all over you and round the clock attention by doctors and nurses. The initial emotions running through me ran the gamut of fear, sadness, anger, regret, and pretty much all the woe is me feeling one gets when beset by a grave illness.

I'd been hospitalized before in 1997 for a burst appendix which further got complicated by peritonitis. That was my first ever hospitalization and I ended up being in that hospital in Burnaby, British Columbia for three weeks to heal. What made that event truly memorable was that my car got stolen overnight in the hospital parking lot that first night. That was like icing on the cake that life's court jesters played on me. I thought that the previous night was memorable enough in the emergency room as I was being prepped for surgery. I was in a tremendous amount of pain lying on that gurney waiting to be brought into the operating room. Then two nurses finally came and they wheeled me in. As I lay down on that gurney side by side on the operating table one of the nurses whispered in my ear. "Can you get on the operating table by yourself? You're too big and heavy for the two of us." I looked at her incredulously at first and then looked at the other nurse who had this wry smile on her face.

I couldn't help but chuckle at this predicament since those two nurses combined were not even close to my body weight of 240 pounds. As I mentioned in my first book I had been battling weight problems since I was a kid. I thought that it was a humorous moment. The last thing I remember as I lay down on the operating table was the mask being putting on my face and I was out. I woke up the next morning groggy and loopy. The nurse came up to me and said, "We have good news and bad news. The good news is we were able to take out your appendix and clean your insides but you have an infection in your abdomen. Oh, and by the way, your car was stolen from our parking lot last night. The good news is that they found it an hour ago. Get some rest and the doctor will update you later." Yes, life is like a box of chocolates.

Fast forward sixteen years later and now I'm here again in the hospital in 2013 facing an even more serious threat to my life. I was thinking to myself that the box of chocolates I got was full of junk because I sure was picking painful chocolate bombs. I was in a dark, sinister, and frightening situation as I could feel my lifeforce slowly draining. Old belief systems programmed into me triggered and I thought I was being punished because I had strayed away from the Catholic faith. Was this God's way of reminding me? It's interesting that fear plays such a major role in religion. I grew up and was educated in Catholic schools all my life. Having read and studied the bible and then being in religion and theology classes all the way up to college was enlightening. Controversial too because of how so many pick and choose what suits them in situations in life.

I had so many thoughts and emotions swirling around in me during that time in the hospital. I had friends visit me and there were priests and nuns also dropping by. My mom had organized a prayer brigade with her network of friends and so did my dad. I come from a deeply devout Catholic family and grew up half-in and half-out the door to that faith. It's like I was a Jekyll and Hyde character. There was a part of me that totally immersed into all the rigid beliefs, ceremonies, and dogma. The other part of me always felt different, always questioning and asking why, but would get submerged down deep into the dark.

I was assessing my situation as I was lying in bed looking at the screen monitoring my vital signs. My heart rate was slowly going down and so was my blood pressure. At one point my heart rate dipped down below forty and my blood pressure was 85/60 and I was scared. I felt so alone even though there were people surrounding me and visiting me. Energetically I was reaching out to Radhaa and Maya The Shaman to help me. Having experienced tremendous success through energy healing the year before and applying the lessons learned from them I knew deep inside to go that route.

We are all energetic beings of light enclosed in this human body which is also a form of energy. We carry electrical charges all over us and our brains and other organs function because of that. We get programmed and stuck on this belief that our existence here on this plane of reality is based on having a human body. I reflected back to 2012 and how Radhaa's and Maya The Shaman's energy healing enabled me to transform my broken down mind and body and overcome obesity and type 2 diabetes. I had to go deep within and start that process again. I had nothing to lose as the doctors at the hospital had no clue what was going on inside of me. They couldn't agree on what was causing this extreme inflammation in my liver and gallbladder. My friends and family members were helpless too and the best thing they did was to pray for me and send me love. Love is the most powerful healing force in this universe. But you have to make that choice to heal and totally believe in it. When you are faced with your mortality so closely there are two choices to make. Forget everything and run or face everything and rise.

Radhaa often said to me that healing is a choice. Those months from November 2011 to October 2012, I was under hers and Maya The Shaman's tutelage. Those lessons and knowledge embedded deeply in me and I had this strong faith that I would overcome this. On my third day in the hospital I woke up startled to see a priest and a nun praying over me. My first thought was he was administering last rites and after the initial shock he said it was an Anointing of the Sick prayer he was doing. He also offered the Act of Confession if I so wanted as I was born and raised a Catholic. I politely declined. I had already made my separation choice in 2011 that I would no longer align or limit myself to that. Many in the same faith find it easy to condemn controversial choices as being blasphemous and that there would be severe repercussions. The beauty of free will as a human is that we can make choices that go against the grain of thinking and believing. I respect and am grateful for that priest and nun who prayed over me that day. That's the universe's way of sending a message that this eternal connection is always there. It doesn't matter the form or delivery method of the package. Love is love.

We are all connected in this vast ever-expanding universe to the very atoms of our being. I would apply the techniques I learned from Radhaa about the power of active breathing through meditation, positive affirmations, talking to my cells, and visualizing and affirming my healing. I was never alone energetically. God, Creator, Source, whatever name we call on externally is within us and all around us.

That third night in the hospital on May 2, 2013 I felt my energetic connection to her, Maya, my mom, my dad, my siblings, my extended family, my friends, and all the others who were praying and sending me love and positive vibes. I concentrated hard and visualized internally and went deep within myself and believed. There was no more fear and I felt the Love energy from everyone permeate into every cell of my being. It's an amazingly beautiful experience mere words cannot properly describe. All I can say is that I felt the life force seeping back into me, albeit slowly.

The next day when I woke up, on May 3, 2013 the doctor came to see me and he was a lot more positive. My liver enzymes had dramatically gone down seemingly overnight and all my other vitals were improving. I had been put through a battery of diagnostic tests and blood draws and urinalysis samples every few hours was getting tiresome for me. I was happy to hear that it had considerably gone down and the so-called sludge that they found in my gallbladder had dissipated. I'll give credit that doctor was still trying to find a way to take my gallbladder out as a precaution. In my mind I wasn't going to give him the satisfaction of adding my gallbladder to his collection. I just told him that I would heal naturally and there would be no need to take it out.

I had a newfound determination that I would let my spirit guide my mind and body to repair and recover. Our bodies have an infinite capacity to heal even with the finite life spans we are given. You just have to connect mind, body, and spirit and develop that mindset of one thriving unit meshing synergistically with each other.

We live in a world where a huge majority live with heads trying to operate as the only functioning processing unit. We forget that we are composed of over seventy trillion cells and each cell is a vital part of the collective.

My immediate motivation was to heal and get out of the hospital. I was horrified by the screams and cries of pain and anguish from the other patients in the wing of that hospital I was in. It was difficult enough to sleep from the pain and discomfort in my body. When you add the emotional assault of fear and pain externally to the internal, your natural instinct is to escape from it.

I continued the internal work of visualization, saying positive affirmations, meditating and talking to my cells, and breathing in love and positivity. A couple of days later on May 5, 2013 I checked out of the hospital, still a bit weak but strong enough to stand up and walk on my own. That was enough.

That metaphorical box of chocolates I was picking up junk from was going to be replaced by one that I would create from the dreams and goals of my true purpose. Create your own reality. Don't accept that life is like a random box of chocolates and is the way the universe works. There is still much beauty out there in this world. You are the master of your own destiny. What you do today and everyday after that becomes your future down the road.

"Whatever the mind of man can conceive and believe, it can achieve."—Napoleon Hill

Chapter 3 -Exhaustion

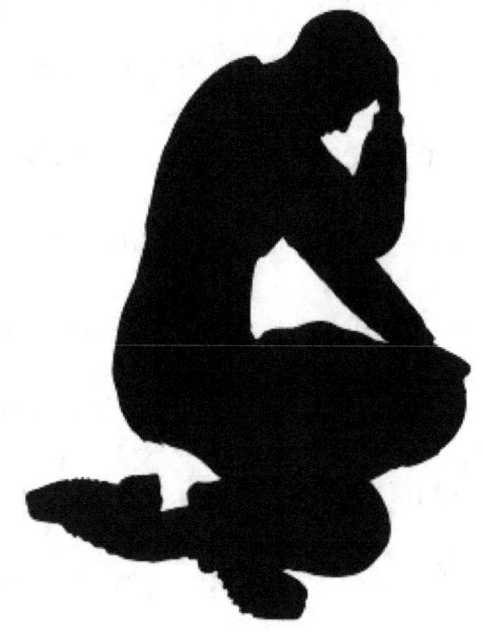

"Awareness is the first step in healing."

- *Dean Ornish*

After 5 days in the hospital I'm finally back home. exhaustion was still permeating throughout my body and my appetite was non-existent. Still, it's better to be at home recuperating than being stuck in that place. I am grateful to everyone at the hospital for doing their best to take care of me. There's still so many questions that need answers and I had to go for weekly blood tests. My liver enzymes were still abnormal but manageable and my jaundice was subsiding. I spent the next few weeks just resting mostly in bed and when I could I would go out for short walks.

I read my hospital discharge report and it was quite extensive. The bottomline was the initial assessment was chronic hepatitis of unknown origin. The most common hepatitis cases everyone is familiar with is types A, B, and C. Mine was still a mystery and so I began to do my own research and implemented rapid changes in my dietary intake. I knew that my liver was quite overloaded and thus needed as much help in ease that burden. I approached it the same way I did when I was on my weight loss and reversing diabetes program the year before. My digestive system needed a lot of healing internally and so I created this nutrition regimen below.

1. Organic power greens (kale, spinach, chard, celery) 2 cups twice a day added to my smoothies and green juices.

2. Eliminating any foods containing any pork, peanuts, wheat, gluten, soy, refined sugars, high fructose corn syrup, and dairy. Eggs

had to be organic and free-range. Also added to the elimination list were processed foods and definitely no more fast-food.

3. Organic homemade bone broth made from grass-fed beef bones, and free-range chicken and turkey bones. I would add Bragg's apple cider vinegar, ginger, garlic, turmeric, himalayan salt, and organic black pepper to the recipe and simmer for 48 hours on low heat. I would sip a cup three times a day with a tablespoon of organic coconut oil or organic ghee to it.

4. I made sure to drink 2 gallons of water daily and would start my mornings with 24 ounces of lukewarm filtered water.

5. My smoothies base would be either organic coconut milk and/or almond milk plus raw organic honey, organic Ceylon cinnamon powder, half a banana, half an avocado, 2 tablespoons organic chia seeds, 1 teaspoon spirulina, and a scoop of vegan protein powder (SAN Rawfusion brand)

6. Maya The Shaman recommended I add zeolite powder for detoxification along with Ashwagandha and Amalaki which are Ayurvedic herbs. My chiropractor also sent me a detoxification powder formula called Cellular Detox.

7. My breakfast staple outside of the smoothies and green juices was organic and gluten-free steel-cut oatmeal with a splash of coconut

milk, 1 tablespoon of organic coconut oil, and a bit of organic coconut sugar.

8. For supplements I resumed my whole-food based multivitamin, B-100 complex, Vitamin C in ester form, natural vitamin E with tocopherols and tocotrienols, 600 mg. of alpha lipoic acid, N-acetyl-cysteine, standardized milk thistle, high EPA/DHA Omega-3 fish oils, and coenzyme Q-10.

I was determined to bring my liver enzymes down to normal. By faithfully incorporating the above regimen with my daily meditations and hour long walks in the park I felt that would bring the liver enzymes down to normal. The physical exhaustion was still lingering but slowly dissipating. Sure enough, by July of 2013 the liver enzymes and bilirubin were back to normal which came as an extreme shock to my gastro-enterologist. He cleared me for travel and going back to the gym too so I excitedly made my plans for going back to Vancouver on August 16, 2013.

Moving back to Canada wasn't something I had planned but what I'd learned about life at that point was to go with the flow and embrace the changes. My wife at that time was going through her own health challenges and our floundering marriage wasn't any help for both of us. We both needed time and space away from each other and I was looking forward to a fresh new start in Vancouver. Everything was seemingly on the upswing and when I arrived in Vancouver on August 16, 2013 I had already outlined my plans.

During my healing period between May 6, 2013 until the day I left I also studied to finally obtain my personal fitness trainer designation from the International Sports Science Association. I passed the exam and got my certificate in July of 2013. By the time I landed in Vancouver I had different career and income options. I hadn't worked out in the gym for three months but I did a lot of walking daily. The only other exercises I could do using my body weight were push-ups, body squats, and walking lunges. My mindset was that I would not allow myself to succumb to the pain and exhaustion. The will to live and thrive was strong and a part of me was angry and still mystified by what had happened.

Upon my arrival in Vancouver it set in motion a whirlwind of movements and events. I enrolled back into the British Columbia Medical Services plan so I could qualify again for health coverage. I interviewed for jobs as a personal fitness trainer at a few different places and I enrolled at the Richmond Olympic Oval so I could work out again.

I fell in love with that Olympic-caliber facility several months before during my previous trip in January of 2013. One of my old friends, Rey Fortaleza, a former Philippine Olympic boxer during the 1976 Montreal Summer Olympics contacted me immediately. He wanted to feature me in my own fitness tv show under his Reyfort Media Group and air it on the Shaw Cable platform. I eagerly accepted his offer and made plans to prepare for production and launch for January of 2014.

Everything seemed to be falling wondrously into place and I felt happy and rejuvenated. I was happy to see all my old friends and it was a special bonding time for me with my parents and sisters. We hadn't seen each other in years and I'm responsible for that disengagement. There was a lot of things inside of me that I needed to acknowledge and come to grips with to heal. The healing sessions the year before with Radhaa and then Maya was the beginning of the healing and unraveling of layers of pain and emotional heartache. It's not easy as a man to come to grips and face emotions unfamiliar yet strangely relieving. Thanks to Radhaa's intuitiveness and compassion I began to tear down the massive walls I had built around myself emotionally.

Vancouver is such a beautiful city and I asked myself why I ever left it. I was also asking myself what if I had not gotten married and had not transferred from GNC Canada to GNC in California? I took a different position and a lower salary to make that happen. So many what ifs swirled around inside of me and I remembered that I had a dream to make it big in America. Now that dream was shattered and I'm picking up the pieces again. Shades of the previous shattered dreams of 1996 from a failed business partnership.

Nevertheless, giving up and crying over spilled milk was not part of my mindset. I viewed this as another opportunity to learn from and make myself even better. I was still exhausted from the hospitalization but I pushed on with my agenda. The first signs that something was not right would soon manifest itself.

I resumed my rigorous workouts at the Richmond Olympic Oval and on my off days I would go to the track in Minoru Park nearby for outdoor activities. I would also go to the Richmond Dyke and walk a couple of hours three times a week. My routine of waking up at 5 am in the morning and do high intensity interval training was back in full swing. I was staying at my sister Maritess' house at the time and I would walk to my parents' apartment a couple of miles away and then walked another mile to the gym. My strength levels for lifting were not the same as they were in 2012 so I pushed myself to get back to that. I had lost more weight from that hospitalization and was hovering around 180-182 pounds. My mom thought I was too skinny now.

Here's a funny tidbit about losing a lot of weight. When I was going through Homeland security checks at the airport the officials would always do a double take looking at my driver's license and passport. I was so much heavier in the picture and the official had to call another official to look at both my license and Canadian passport. They needed to make sure I was the same person.

The first ominous sign that something was not fully healed was after an intense deadlifting morning workout session in September of 2013. I felt nauseous and dizzy after that and I was wondering if I had done too much. An hour later after that I was taking a hot shower at my parents' apartment when I suddenly started quivering and shaking and I felt so hot. I stumbled out of the shower, dried off, and collapsed in a heap on my parents' bed shaking uncontrollably. My mom checked my temperature which had skyrocketed and I was burning up. She and my dad were concerned and I said I must have caught some kind of bug. I refused to take any fever and pain relief medication and the fever soon gave way to a bout of feeling extremely cold. Mom bundled me up in a thick blanket as I shivered and shaked. A few hours later everything subsided like it had never happened and I felt fine.

My thoughts were racing and I started to ask myself if the workout and the pre-workout supplements I had resumed taking were responsible. I monitored myself the next few weeks while still using the same pre-workout supplements on top of my regular supplement protocol. The fever incident didn't happen and I chalked it up to a 24-hour kind of bug. I was still on the same regimen of nutrition I outlined at the start of this chapter and I felt great. Then another incident occurred a few weeks later when I woke up with my upper lip all swollen up like I had gotten stung or bitten by something. Or maybe it was something I ate.

I was retracing what I had eaten the night before and I remembered I had eaten a small box of blackberries. I love berries of all kinds especially blueberries, raspberries, strawberries, and blackberries. I had been regularly adding them to my smoothies for years and never had any problems. I made sure they were also organic and washed so I was confused. I went through my sister's kitchen pantry and reading all the labels of the food I had purchased. Was there something I was reacting to now and had manifested in my more sensitive state since the hospitalization? I'm proficient at reading labels and identifying ingredients and I saw nothing amiss in what I had purchased. Mystified, I kept close scrutiny and awareness of my internal conditions.

A few more weeks passed with no more incidents and heading into November all systems were go. I made some new friends that were going to be part of my show and it turned out that we were going to produce two shows. The first would be my fitness show called Fitness with Mike and the second show would be a show about life as a new immigrant in Canada called The Big Shift. My new friends Gigi Grey-Ricarse, Crisanta Sampang, and Raymond Maghirang would be part of that show. We were all excited and we were having weekly meetings writing out our shows' scripts and planning the different location shoots. I also got featured in my friend Rey Fortaleza's newspaper

Philippine Asian New Today for the October 31, 2013 edition. Yes, life seemed so much on the upswing.

November 10, 2013 would be another historical day and it would be the beginning of a new path and evolution for me. I woke up that morning to intense pain in my upper abdomen. It was a far more intense pain than before and it was excruciating. I inspected myself all over and didn't see any yellow spots indicating jaundice. I looked in the mirror and didn't see any yellow in my eyes.

I remembered the previous events from the past couple of months and this time I said to myself I would nip this in the bud. I walked to the Richmond hospital emergency room that afternoon after the pain wouldn't go away. This would be another pivotal event and more revelations would soon come.

I was lying again on an emergency room bed having blood drawn and urine samples taken for tests. The results came back a few hours later and it showed my liver enzymes were highly elevated again to 15 times the normal. I had already explained my story and previous hospitalization in Anaheim to the attending physician. He looked at me with a serious gaze and he said I wasn't going anywhere. I'm back in the hospital again and I was distraught and saddened.

My parents came to check on me that night and the doctor told them I would have to be admitted in. Deep inside though, I knew something was going on and now it was fully blown out into the open. The mystery had to be resolved and I steeled myself for a much harder and longer battle.

The fear of the unknown triggered and activated again in me that warrior mode that I had summoned several months ago when I was first hospitalized. I prepared myself for a much longer and harder battle.

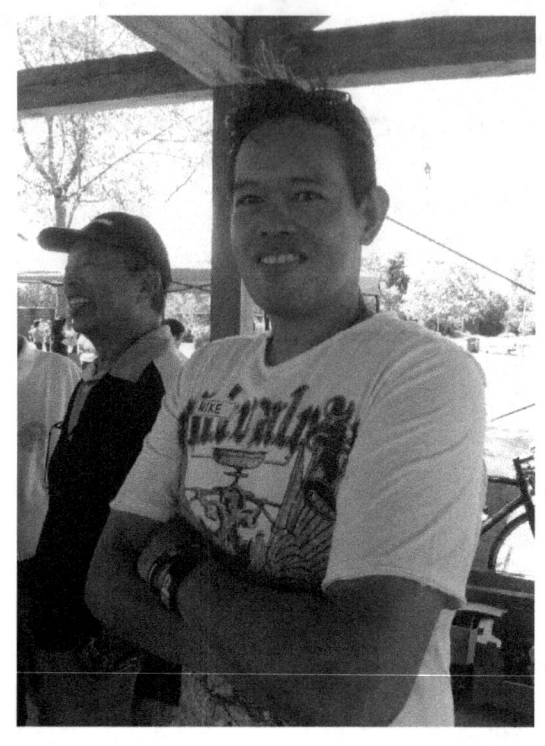

"You've done it before and you can do it now. See the positive possibilities. Redirect the substantial energy of your frustration and turn it into, positive, effective, unstoppable determination."

- Ralph Marston

Chapter 4- I Know My Enemy

"What matters is this: Being fearless of failure arms you to break the rules. In doing so, you may change the culture and just possibly, for a moment, change life itself".- Malcolm Mclaren

Faced with my mortality once again in less than six months there were so many thoughts and emotions were roiling inside me. There was a bit of fear creeping in but the emotions bubbling up to the surface were those of anger and frustration.

Why was this happening now that I had already made the transition to a healthy lifestyle? I enjoyed a year of life with unfettered energy, focus, and becoming happier with myself. Why now? What lessons are forthcoming?

The room I was in at the Richmond Hospital was shared with three other seriously ill patients all much older than me. Once again, I had tubes and needles stuck in me and the familiar screen monitoring my vital signs beside me too. The big difference with this second round in a hospital was that my energy levels weren't as low but the pain was more excruciating in my abdominal area. My stomach region felt like there was some kind of blockage and my liver area was throbbing. I wasn't jaundiced so I took that as a positive. The first few days showed that the elevated liver enzymes and bilirubin levels were at least ten times the normal range.

I once again had to explain to my new Canadian doctors what happened to me when I was hospitalized in Anaheim. To make it easier I suggested to request all my medical records from Anaheim Regional Memorial. While waiting for the records to be sent I would have to endure blood samples drawn four times a day. I asked the doctor how long I would have to stay in confinement and he said to just be patient. He wanted to get to the bottom of this mysterious affliction too. The blood tests confirmed again I had no hepatitis A, B, or C and that was a relief.

The first week in the hospital was a test of patience. Between the nighttime screams and crying of my fellow patients and nurses waking me up at 3 am to draw several tubes of blood I just focused on what I learned from Radhaa about meditation. I would focus on my breathing and visualizations and channel my emotions and thoughts inward. I had my iPhone beside me so I tuned into healing music videos. Healing sound frequencies are so soothing and calming and it transported me to another dimension of peace and love.

My cousin Patrick would drop by to visit me after work and would bring me over magazines to read. I'm so grateful to him for being one of the few to visit me in the hospital. He knew how much I loved to read and he brought me a lot to read. I'm a voracious reader and have been since I was young. I liked keeping my mind active and informed to what was happening. It's a habit ingrained in me by my parents and I'm grateful I developed that habit to be a wide reader. Aside from the magazines I used my iPhone to go on the Internet and do my own research. I was determined to find clues to this unknown condition.

During the day the nurses would encourage me to go walk around the hospital floor and get some exercise. I was still in a lot of pain and getting up was not easy. They were tough but loving and their daily encouragement was motivating and helpful to my morale. One of them recognized me from the article written about me by the Philippine Asian News Today. She said my story was inspiring and that I shouldn't give up. Positive reinforcement does wonders for a tired body and mind.

Days stretched into three weeks and my liver enzymes were slowly improving and dropping and I couldn't wait to be discharged. The records from Anaheim Regional Medical had not arrived and I was getting anxious, antsy, and irritable why it took so long. My appetite wasn't back to normal and my stomach was still sensitive. I would subsist on beef broth, chicken soup, vegetable soup, apples, and bananas. My parents would bring me a box of Filipino steamed rice cakes called puto which was my childhood favorite. That was the only comfort food I could tolerate without having my stomach explode into a paroxysm of painful activity.

I kept applying the meditation and visualization lessons I learned from Radhaa and Maya and found inner calm and peace amidst the stormiest time of my life. Being in bed for so long will make anyone feel bored, irritable, and anxious. The best remedy is movement and I would make it a point to get up and walk around the hospital floor and do laps. I wasn't shuffling around anymore unlike the first week and the pain was manageable. I also got over the initial embarrassment of walking around in a hospital gown with my butt exposed. I was observing everything going on around me and using all my senses. My neighbors in the room I was in were quiet for the most part except for this one guy who was in a lot of pain and always moaning and crying.

The doctors and the nurses were trying to help him out but there was a language barrier. I knew he was Chinese and in his early fifties and the Chinese nurse assigned to him was trying to get him to talk. It turns out he had been living in Canada for the last twenty-five years as a dishwasher. The sad thing is he never learned English and lived and worked in isolation. He had no family or even friends around to call on and the nurse kept asking him why he never learned English and make new connections. I can only imagine how lonely it must have been for him to live like that for twenty-five years.

Being in a hospital really brings an up close and personal reminder about the circle of life, sickness, and death. I had been there for three weeks in that hospital room and witness to a revolving door of patients. Some were moved around while some transitioned on. The unmistakable flat-line sounds of the monitors during the night were a stark reminder of my mortality. At first, I was afraid of hearing that someone had passed on. I kept on doing my meditations and prayers and I felt the presence of the angels and spirit guides. That practice kept me at peace and provided joy and happiness during the suffering.

I didn't consider myself as or be labeled and limited to being called a Catholic. I still believe in God, Creator, Source Energy, and all the other versions of light energy extending from that. This is my journey and my path of my own free will and I am happy and secure with it.

My parents would come over daily and pray over me daily in their own way using the holy rosary. They respected my decision about going on my own way and disentangling myself from a religion I was thrust into without the benefit of informed choice. I'm a spiritual being inhabiting a human body living and experiencing life in this plane of reality. I knew there was a purpose for what was going on inside of me and with that, learning to just go with the flow of life. It's not an easy path and the feelings and emotions inside of me reminded me of that. The burning question I had was this, "What is this mysterious condition that no one has answers for and when will the answer be revealed?"

After three and a half weeks of being in the hospital and still no answers after numerous tests, my condition was determined to be good enough for me to be released. The liver enzymes and bile levels had dramatically gone down to near normal and that was a huge relief. The doctors were still waiting for my lab results from the hospital in Anaheim and told me that they would let me know once they received it. The instructions were to go to the lab nearby for weekly blood tests and coordinate with my family doctor. My parents suggested I stay with them at their place to rest and recover. When love is offered don't let your pride get in the way. Be open to receiving the love that is offered to you unconditionally.

While waiting for my doctors to determine what was going on inside of me I focused on the other aspects. I analyzed my diet and my fitness programs again and made some decisions to help de-stress and heal my digestive system. I found in my Google Drive a copy of an old metabolic test from 2008 done by Metametrix. This company provides metabolic, toxicant, and nutritional testing to help identify the underlying causes of chronic disease. I had this metabolic profile test done while I was an independent contractor for Designs for Health and I completely forgot about the contents of the report.

Metametrix IgG Food Antibodies and Celiac Profile was the test that was done on me back then. The Allergix IgG4 antibody is related to "delayed" or non-atopic food reactions that exacerbate or contribute to many different health problems. Simultaneous high levels of many IgG4 food-specific antibodies are generally associated with intestinal hyperpermeability. This profile measures the IgG4 levels in serum that react to 90 different foods, including commonly eaten foods such as corn, milk, egg, and wheat. A food reaction patient guide is provided with each test result. This guide was what I was reading and trying to understand in detail.

Even if these test results were from 2008 the information contained in the report were still viable. I don't know why I didn't take these results more seriously and implemented it back then. This report took on a much more dramatic importance as the results showed many different food sensitivities ranging from mild, moderate, and severe. The most severe reactions for me were from pork and dairy products from cow's milk. Next in line for the moderate was grapefruit, peanuts, almonds, and wheat. The mild sensitivities were from sesame, blackberries, blueberries, strawberries, and raspberries. It was all starting to make sense to me when I read the report. My hypothesis was that perhaps my liver and digestive system got compromised and severely irritated by my continued consumption of those particular foods. This kind of test is not one that a regular medical doctor recommends for a patient. From my experience in working with integrative and holistic health practitioners this was the kind of testing they would recommend to their patients to address health conditions modern Western medicine was not open to.

Right then and there I made a choice to avoid and eliminate all those foods listed and took it a few steps further. I'd go raw, vegan, non-GMO, organic, gluten-free, and avoid anything processed. I was determined to heal myself no matter what. The doctors couldn't help me much when it came to the nutrition aspect. They simply told me to resume eating a normal balanced diet. I've come to expect that kind of response from those in the medical profession that are not into integrative medicine. I was going to rely on my own initiative and knowledge of nutrition and exercise to carry me through this.

While I was waiting for my lab tests to arrive from Anaheim I focused on moving forward. My doctor in Canada gave me the okay to resume light activities at the Richmond Olympic Oval. I wrote down my diet and supplement plan to begin the healing process internally. My doctors didn't believe in supplements and one of them had a theory that it was the supplements that affected my liver and gallbladder. But there was nothing definitive to prove that seeing that there were so many other factors they were taking into consideration. At least this doctor was open enough to nutritional supplements and didn't tell me to stop taking them. This particular doctor I came to highly respect not just for his open mindedness to my protocol. He also was also regularly working out at the same gym I went to. At least here was one practitioner that took care of his body too.

Working out in the gym was therapy not just for my body but my mind and spirit as well. Visualization and focusing on deep breathing during the exercises was key to numbing the pain and discomfort I still felt inside of me. My gut was highly inflamed inside and I didn't need to have a health professional tell me that. Since I started on this process of natural healing when I began my weight loss journey I've learned to be more attuned to my body on a deeper level. I had to transmute the pain and exhaustion and channel it into an effective workout session.

Aside from the gym I would go on long two-hour walks daily either at Minoru Park or around the dyke outside of Richmond Olympic Oval. I did this routine faithfully and willed myself to get up early in the morning at 6 am and get to the gym and then go for my walks at night. I had to keep my mind preoccupied and not get caught up in worrying. I focused as well on looking at all the blessings I had in my life. It was a special time that December since I'd be spending Christmas with my sisters and my parents in Canada. We hadn't been together for over a decade and this would be our first Christmas holiday celebration together. As I said earlier before I'm not what you would call a deeply religious person for many years but I valued the family time with them. That was enough and living in the moment was truly special.

After almost two months of waiting my doctor's office finally called and scheduled my appointment for January 27, 2014. During that period of healing time I took on a couple of gigs as an independent personal trainer and as a natural foods broker for Ecoideas. I wasn't the type to just lay in bed all day. Even if I was feeling weak, in pain, and nauseous from the ordeal I kept my focus and would not allow myself to wallow in self-pity.

January 27, 2014 – this fateful day is forever marked in my calendar. I took the Skytrain to the downtown Vancouver office of my liver specialist.

There was a combination of apprehension, nervousness, and confidence I was feeling on the way there. I kept telling myself I would just go with the flow and trust in the universe.

I arrived at the medical center and was promptly ushered in to my doctor's office. He walks in after a few minutes with a fairly thick file folder which I assumed was my file. After the usual cordial greetings between us I asked him, "So what's the verdict Doc? Have you found out what's going on inside of me? Just give it to me and not sugarcoat things. I can handle this."

He looks at me seriously and he says, "Mike, after an exhaustive analysis of your records from California and our own rigorous testing and consulting with the best panel of specialists here in British Columbia I'm afraid that you have a rare autoimmune condition called Autoimmune Hepatitis and it's incurable."

I was stunned upon hearing it and I gathered myself quickly to respond, "Autoimmune hepatitis? I have an autoimmune disorder that's incurable? How bad is it?"

He replied, "You have Stage 3-4 fibrosis with significant scarring in your liver and left untreated you will need a liver transplant. Thankfully you don't have cirrhosis or cancer but you're basically at the closest point to it with your liver function perilously close to 5%. There is no medical treatment that will cure this type of hepatitis but we can stave off further attacks by your body through immune-suppressing medication. It's fairly safe and we will monitor you over the next three months and see how your body responds to this treatment. I'm really sorry."

I knew about and was familiar with immune-suppressing drugs and I wanted to confirm with him the side effects.

Me: "Please tell me more about the side-effects of this treatment. I know that with all these drugs there are side-effects that come with it. You are referring to corticosteroids right?"

Doctor: "You are correct. We recommend several drugs Imuran, Azathioprine, and Urso over the next three months. The side-effects are that you will experience bloating, gain weight, and exhibit symptoms of a Type 2 Diabetic. That is our recommendation."

Me: "Basically you're recommending that I go take these drugs and go back to being obese and type 2 Diabetic? What the hell kind of option is that? I just lost over 100 pounds in 2012 and got off all the diabetes medications in 2011 and started enjoying a life full of energy and happiness. Who in their right mind wants to go back to that? Hell no, I am not going back to that! I'm sorry, that's just not an option I will take. I respect and appreciate you and all the wonderful doctors who have been helping me. I don't accept the word impossible and incurable. I believe I'm possible and I'm curable and I will find a way! I will work with you and your team to monitor my blood tests and my liver's condition but I will not take any more drugs!"

Doctor: "I understand and respect how you feel and I won't stand in your way. All I ask is that you continue to go have your blood tested every week for the next three months so we can assess your progress. I also want to make it very clear that we will document and record here that you are not accepting our treatment recommendations. You do understand and appreciate that right?"

Me: "Absolutely! I'll work with you and I'll show everyone that impossible is just an opinion. I want copies of my medical records showing this diagnosis and I will be the first one to heal from it. Thank you for everything."

With that said I got up and left his office and took the elevator back down. So many thoughts were racing through my head and my heart was pounding so loud in my head. When the elevator reached the floor level I stepped out and I burst into tears and started sobbing. I knew I was heading into uncharted waters and believing in hope and faith to carry me through. I was afraid and I was angry but now I knew the name of my enemy. Time to buckle up, strap down, and get to work!

Chapter 5 – I Will Live

"A lot of people say they want to get out of pain, and I'm sure that's true, but they aren't willing to make healing a high priority. They aren't willing to look inside to see the source of their pain in order to deal with it." -Lindsay Wagner

After the initial shock of the official diagnosis and my breakdown in the office lobby I felt a strange sense of relief wash over me. I was grateful I finally knew it was autoimmune hepatitis I was up against. Now I could begin creating a path towards healing this incurable disease.

What is autoimmune hepatitis? In medical terms it is a rare chronic disease of unknown cause highlighted by continuous inflammation of the liver cells and necrosis with a propensity to progress to cirrhosis. At the time of my first hospitalization at Anaheim Regional hospital from April 29 to May 6, 2013 the official medical report showed I had chronic hepatitis of unknown cause. They couldn't pinpoint it as autoimmune hepatitis at the time even when presented with the symptoms of jaundice, fever, and liver tenderness. Later on I found out through my own research that some patients with this condition develop symptoms of chronic liver disease while others rapidly progress to acute liver failure. The doctors were baffled how my body was able to rapidly bring down the extremely high liver enzymes in just a few days. One thing they did tell me was that because I was in excellent physical condition that it most likely saved me. I reflect on that and am grateful for the transformation journey I took a couple of years before that to lose over 107 pounds and reverse type 2 diabetes.

I exhibited many of the classic symptoms of autoimmune hepatitis which included the following:

- Fatigue (I felt so drained all the time.)

- Upper abdominal discomfort (this was a real pain and I had to endure that daily)

- Myalgia (muscle pain that I first attributed to my regular workouts but didn't subside)

- Diarrhea

- Skin Rashes

- Chest pain from pleuritis

- Jaundice

My lab findings from the two hospitalizations in Anaheim and Vancouver further confirmed it with the following:

- Elevated serum aminotransferase levels (1.5-50 times reference values)

- Elevated serum immunoglobulin levels, primarily immunoglobulin G (IgG)

- Mild to moderately elevated serum bilirubin and alkaline phosphatase – In 80-90% of patients; a sharp increase in the alkaline phosphatase values during the course of autoimmune disease may reflect the development of primary sclerosing cholangitis (PSC) or the onset of hepatocellular carcinoma as a complication of cirrhosis

- Seropositive results for antinuclear antibodies (ANAs), smooth-muscle antibodies (SMAs), or liver-kidney microsomal type 1 (LKM-1) or anti–liver cytosol 1 (anti-LC1) antibodies

- Hypoalbuminemia and prolongation of prothrombin time – Markers of severe hepatic synthetic dysfunction, which may be observed in active disease or decompensated cirrhosis.

The liver biopsy that was done and analyzed again by the specialist team in Vancouver confirmed it.

The typical course of management of autoimmune hepatitis for the last 3 decades has been the use of corticosteroids, alone or in combination with another drug, azathioprine. This was the recommended course of treatment by my doctor in Vancouver which I refused. Brave or stupid? I just had this firm belief and conviction that I would heal myself.

My research showed that with autoimmune hepatitis relapse occurs in 50% of patients within 6 months of treatment withdrawal and in 80% of patients within 3 years of treatment. Reinstating the original treatment regimen usually induced another remission; however, relapse commonly recurred after a second attempt at terminating therapy. Patients who relapsed twice require indefinite therapy with either prednisone or azathioprine. These facts didn't present a comforting picture of my survival yet I remained undaunted.

I remained undaunted while fear would sometimes fuel angst and anger throughout my healing period. I talked to my parents and my sisters about my decision to go at it on a natural and holistic level. They respected my decision and supported me all the way. There's two ways you can define how you approach fear. Face everything and rise or forget everything and run. All my life I've never run away from any challenges presented to me and this challenge was going to be my Mount Everest. Was I afraid? Hell, yes! Was I going to run away?

Hell, no! I was going to make my stand and make the impossible possible on my own terms.

I'm grateful that I accumulated so much knowledge, experience, and wisdom over the years about nutrition, diet, exercise, and the incorporation of spiritual principles which I learned from Radhaa and Maya The Shaman. It provided me with a solid foundation to create a healing protocol to turn back this progressive and deadly disease.

Putting together a healing protocol that is complete and all-encompassing means digging deep and integrate mind, body, and spirit. The typical Western approach to treatment is to find ways to fix the symptoms with a pill or medicine of some kind. I knew from experience that I blindly accepted this philosophy for the most part of my life. In my first book I AM Enough- Healing A Broken Body I shared my story about how I lost weight and reversed type 2 Diabetes. More importantly, it was the mental and spiritual lessons that truly set me on the path towards an irreversible transformation.

To fight this disease I would have to call on the investigative and instinctive techniques to find those needles in a haystack and put them all together. The mind and spirit cannot forever sustain the body if the foundation of nutrients necessary for biological function are not optimal. Contrary to what the so-called experts in America say about the safety of the Western food supply and its highly processed nature I scoffed at this. Why? Look around you and you can see the physical evidence along with the fact that diabetes, obesity, cancer, and heart disease rates have gone up in correlation with the population. No medicine can fix the massive addiction to over-indulgence and unhealthy relations with food that is over-processed and filled with empty calories.

I shared in chapter three that I switched over to a whole food plant-based, dairy-free and gluten-free lifestyle in 2014 as part of my initial protocol. My upper abdominal discomfort was so severe that almost any food I ate caused excruciating pain. While I was recuperating at my parent's place and subsequently at my sister Maritess' I initiated that nutrition protocol and made sure that all the vegetables, fruits, nuts, grains and seeds I consumed were to be organic and non-GMO as much as possible. The first few months of 2014 I found my stomach could only handle certain cooked foods like organic oatmeal, chia and flax seeds, and this traditional Filipino rice cake called puto. To supplement my protein intake I found three brands of vegan protein powder, Sunwarrior, Reliv Pro Vantage, and SAN's Rawfusion that my digestive system had no problems handling.

The fatigue during those early months of 2014 was debilitating and I had some really bad days wherein I was just in bed. I knew I had to muster some kind of physical activity otherwise my muscles would wither and atrophy even further. I would drag myself out and go for a nightly walk at the track oval across my parents' apartment. My goal was to do at least twenty laps around that oval daily and do walking lunges the length of the soccer field. I made that commitment and set my mind to it and just did it. I also made a commitment to myself to go to the gym at the Richmond Olympic Oval and lift weights twice a week.

Here's the thing about exercise, it will heal and rejuvenate you. Once that blood gets flowing after five to ten minutes of brisk activity it produces those endorphins that change not just your physical disposition but your mental one as well. The weightlifting also helped my body naturally produce growth hormones and keep my muscles and bones strong. Healing is a choice like my dear friend Radhaa would say to me before and I took that to heart. You have to make that choice and do the work yourself. No one can do it for you.

The last part of my daily routine was to meditate and journal before I went to sleep and before I got out of bed. We often neglect this key aspect because we prioritize our lives with the hustle and bustle of daily life along with the temptations and desires of watching television and immersing ourselves on the Internet and social media. We all have twenty-four hours in a day and it is what you prioritize that determines the quality of your life in that day. Meditation and journaling was something I learned from my spiritual coaches Radhaa and Maya The Shaman and I'm so grateful to them for that. Radhaa shared with me so many resources on meditation on YouTube and Soundcloud that calmed, soothed my soul, and helped heal my mind and body through the frequencies of the music I listened to. I learned how to be actively purposeful in my breathing for meditation from my healing sessions with Radhaa and Maya The Shaman back in 2011 and 2012. Radhaa's online school Goddess Code Academy and her unique, powerful, and effective modality The Goddess Code Activations™ along with Maya The Shaman's Lemurian Code Healing are an excellent addition to a healthy holistic life.

To round off and complement my nutrition program I tweaked my nutrition supplement protocol. There are those in the medical field that would question this and some believe that by eating a balanced diet one does not need to supplement. As I said earlier, the evidence around us shows people are getting fatter and sicker even with all these so-called advances in modern medicine. More and more people are turning towards cleaner organic foods and demanding change and accountability from the companies that we have trusted for our health. Go to any grocery and supermarket in Canada and the United States and you will see an ever-growing selection of organic foods.

For those living with autoimmune disease and especially with this autoimmune hepatitis I cannot emphasize how important it is to begin your healing through the food and drink you ingest. With a compromised liver and digestive system the body needs some extra help to begin healing inside. One of my old standby books for natural healing is Prescription for Nutritional Healing by Phyllis A. Balch. I've been using it as my ultimate resource and it has never failed me.

I also do research on the Internet on my favorite alternative medicine websites of Dr. Joseph Mercola, Dr. Weil, Dr. Josh Axe, Dr. Mark Hyman, Dr. Burton Berkson and Dr. Neal Barnard. Through my research from all these sources I came up with my own nutritional supplement protocol specific not just to the autoimmune hepatitis but also managing type 2 Diabetes and taking into consideration my fitness regimen.

This next chapter I'll put it all together and show how the impossible can be made possible. Oh, one more thing, by April 2014 my liver enzymes went back to normal and have remained so to this day in 2018. Believe in yourself! Anything is possible!

Chapter 6 – I Am Healing

"It is during our darkest moments that we must focus to see the light."

—Aristotle Onassis

This period of time was indeed a darkest moment of my life. Even as I put on a brave face externally to the outside world inside I was a cauldron of seething, raging and volcanic energy. My spiritual coach Radhaa of Goddess Code Academy(www.goddesscodeacademy.com) told me back in 2012 that healing is an ongoing process and there would be more layers that would have to be shed moving forward. Prophetic words indeed and I'm grateful that she didn't sugarcoat anything at all. Because of her I learned to go through life and not just around it. I detailed in my first book how she helped me complete my transformation. Now in this book I get to apply the timeless lessons she instilled in me that would help discern and put it all together to save my life. It's truly about connecting the mind, body, and spirit as one the way it is supposed to be. To achieve this connection means going deep inward while providing the right mental and physical nutrition and exercise externally.

My physical state in 2014 was like that of a severely damaged computer system. My liver was in dire straits and along with that my digestion. I was in constant pain yet I refused to take any pain medication anymore. No more of that damn naproxen, Tylenol, and Advil that I used to pop like candy when I was younger. I was told they were safe and I blindly trusted that and it almost killed me. I was angry and looking for someone and anyone to blame at that point. The more I found out about my condition and what contributed to it the angrier I became. I zeroed in on how I was raised and brought up as a baby. I found out I was only breastfed and was on baby formula as early as two months old. That was the advice given to my mom and she followed the doctors. I grew up as a sickly baby because of that advice. In my first book I outlined how the other factors specifically with the excessive consumption of sugar and processed foods in conjunction with my genetic predisposition of having a weak liver contributed to my current state of dysfunctional health. I was mad at my parents for not knowing better and for giving me so much toxic food and contributing to my unhealthy relationship with food and myself. That was my lowest point emotionally in 2014 even as my parents were taking care of me. I would swing back and forth between forgiveness and gratitude to anger and resentment. It's natural to feel the way I felt and it's important to own all those feelings as well.

The path towards healing required me to go deep into the shadows of my damaged self. I recognized that it wasn't just my body that needed healing. I needed to heal mentally and emotionally and spiritually. I had to be patient, persistent, passionate, courageous, dedicated, and committed to the path of natural healing I chose. Most of all, I needed to be willing to go into the darkness and accept it as a part of my complete existence. Once in the darkness I had to find a way to let that light shine in there.

My body was highly inflamed inside especially my liver and digestive system and I had to start putting out the fire. You're not going to heal by popping a pill or drink a potion that just masks and temporarily relieves the damage. We rely too much on the brainwashing here that you can solve all your health problems with pharmaceuticals. There's a time and place for that but we have abused it and used it as a crutch. The path starts with nutrition and here's what I put together that year.

Nutrition- Food and Drink

- Eliminate all processed foods. If you want to live and to heal properly you're going to have to quit eating junk food and fast food. Same goes for your daily fix of drinks loaded with sugar and hydrogenated fats. Yes, that means no sodas, none of those hydration and vitamin drinks loaded with caffeine and sugar. Even those fruit juices that innocently look healthy are also stealth bombers detrimental to your health. No more of those pesticide-laden, sugar loaded, boxes of cereal you think is part of a healthy breakfast.

- Start reading labels. Take responsibility for and own and commit to your healing program. Eliminate anything that has high fructose corn syrup, hydrogenated fats, artificial sweeteners, artificial flavorings, artificial colors and dyes. Limit your consumption of added sugars to 25 to 35 grams daily.

This doesn't mean you have to go exclusively to Whole Foods, Sprouts, and other health store chains. Today's modern North American supermarkets and grocery chains have expanded their selections so you can find healthy organic food without losing your whole paycheck.

- Drink 3 to 4 liters daily. Personally, my own intake was 6 to 8 liters of alkaline water. Start off your day the moment you get up with 16 to 24 ounce glasses of pure filtered water with either a couple of teaspoons of organic apple cider vinegar or if you prefer with lemon juice. You're going to be eliminating all the toxics that have built up and taken residence in your fat cells. Limit or eliminate consumption of water from any plastic bottle that contains BPA or Bisphenol-A. This toxic lining found in many plastic bottles and in canned goods is a carcinogen and also introduces xenoestrogens that wreak havoc inside your body. For a comprehensive understanding of xenoestrogens that are beyond the scope of my book I refer you to the book The Toxin Solution by Dr. Joseph Pizzorno. It will be an eye-opener for sure. I was already familiar with the hidden synthetic estrogens in our food supply and environment and made a conscious effort since 2014 to avoid them.

- Eliminate dairy and gluten from your diet. Today's modern dairy products are loaded with growth hormone, antibiotics and all sorts of chemicals that really contribute to the inflammation inside. The animals that sacrifice their lives to produce and provide our food live a horrific life full of abuse and fear. We are all energetic beings and guess what happens when you ingest food with a low vibration? It brings your vibration down as well and contributes to the dysfunction of your body and mind. I found that when I eliminated all dairy from my diet that I had immediate relief from chest congestion, mucus production, elimination of skin rashes and diarrhea, and most of all, from severe abdominal distress.

Secondly, when I started to eliminate any product with gluten specifically wheat the bloating and stomach distress I was experiencing subsided. Not totally but enough that I could get by the day. Thankfully there are a lot of gluten-free options now available in stores. Dining out is more of a challenge though so you have to be really careful which places you go have a bite. There are lots of hidden gluten-containing foods and here's a laundry list to avoid as much as possible:

- malt/malt flavoring

- packaged soups

- commercial bullion and broths

- cold cuts

- French fries (often dusted with flour before freezing)

- processed cheese

- mayonnaise

- ketchup

- malt vinegar

- soy sauce and teriyaki sauces

-salad dressings

- imitation crab meat

- bacon

- egg substitute

- tabbouleh

- sausage

- non-dairy creamer

- fried vegetables/tempura

- gravy

- marinades

- canned baked beans

- cereals

- commercially prepared chocolate milk

- breaded foods

- fruit fillings and puddings

- hot dogs

- ice cream

- root beer

- energy bars

- trail mix

- syrups

- seitan

- wheatgrass

- instant hot drinks

- flavored coffees and teas blue cheeses

- vodka

- wine coolers

- meatballs, meatloaf communion wafers

- veggie burgers

- roasted nuts

- beer

- oats (unless certified GF)

- oat bran (unless certified GF)

I looked at this long list and I realized just how much hidden gluten was in the food I was consuming. I was discussing this with my sister Maritess and we were trying to figure out what I could eat. Those first few months in 2014 was trying my patience and my will to heal. Not only was I feeling weak from the autoimmune condition I was afraid to eat anything beyond oatmeal, rice cakes made from rice flour, vegetable soup(ginger, garlic, celery, carrots, kale, spinach), fruit and veggie smoothies(made with almond or coconut milk, fresh or frozen fruit like blueberries, mangoes, raspberries, peaches, bananas, blackberries, moringa powder, almond butter, kale, spinach, chard, vegan protein powder, chia and flax seeds, coconut oil).

My sister shares the same passion for cooking and baking like me took it upon herself to create a healthy, nutrient-dense, and delicious cookie which would make it easy for me to get the nutrition I needed. She bought all organic ingredients and created a vegan, gluten-free, nut-free variety of cookies and muffins that helped me get back on my feet. Not only did it get me back on my feet it helped me mentally, emotionally, and spiritually. Food made with love heals compared to a soul-less production made in a factory.

Here's what one recipe looks like:

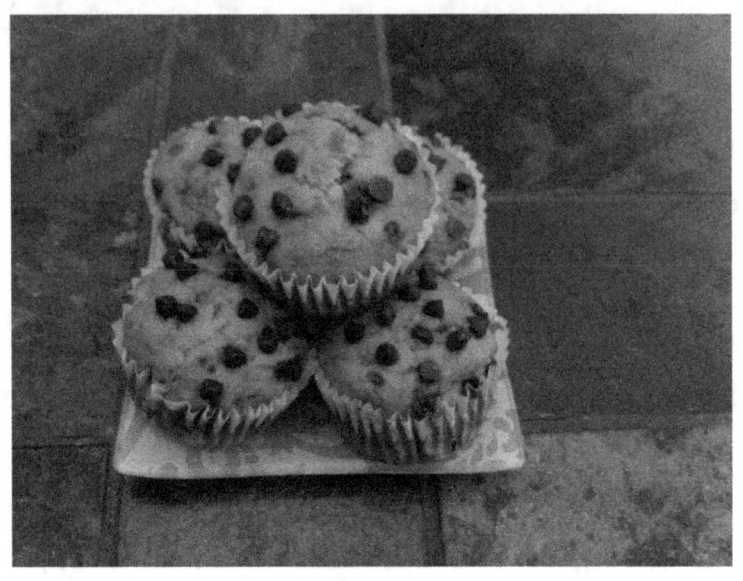

My main food choices during this time of healing my gut and my liver were very limited initially but I discovered a whole new world later on with vegetables and fruits, seeds, and nuts. Limits are truly a creation of the mind and the abundance of blessings from the earth are boundless. It was easy for me to create my own plant-based recipes for salads, smoothies, and baked goods. Another nugget of wisdom I will share with you is that you must shift towards a growth mindset and an open mind to possibilities. A closed mind that lives inside a rigid belief system limits you and hurts you.

I made a choice to limit my consumption of animal products as my healing progressed and when I did I made sure they were organic, free-range, grass-fed, pasture-raised, cage-free, environments. I also started introducing home-made bone broths made from beef and chicken bones simmered for over 48 hours with healing and savory herbs like turmeric, ginger, garlic, rosemary, oregano, Himalayan salt, and black pepper. All organic is what I highly recommend all the way to the spices.

By the time spring of 2014 rolled around my blood tests were all normal for liver enzymes. My doctors were pleasantly surprised on both sides of the border and happy that what I was doing was working. I was just happy to be able to be able to travel back and forth, work out, meditate, make new friendships, and re-establish old networks in Vancouver. My nutrition regimen involved the use of dietary supplements which I discuss next.

My daily diet was also infused with organic superfoods like moringa powder, chia and flax seeds, spirulina and chlorella, turmeric, ginger, garlic, cinnamon, coconut oil and coconut milk, quinoa, and cacao powder. One of my favorite drinks was a warm mug of golden milk which I made with coconut milk, ginger, turmeric, cinnamon and black pepper. It was a potent liver cleanser and soothing for my digestive system.

My Nutrition Supplement Protocol

My core foundation started with combining supplements that would enable me to optimize the assimilation of the food I consumed and help heal me inside, help me recover, reduce inflammation, and improve my mental focus, clarity, and mood. My experience and knowledge about supplements from my years working for GNC and then as an independent health educator for integrative health practitioners enable me to create a healing protocol that really worked for me. Will it work for you and heal your autoimmune condition? I'm not a doctor and I can't guarantee all of this works for you so before you implement my program it's best to consult with a medical professional. This was just a part of the complete holistic mind, body, and spirit approach I took. Many people make the mistake of picking and selecting only from a physical standpoint and neglect the mind and spirit. Trust in the complete process and commit to it like I did.

I provided my doctors with a list of all these supplements I took and even though they were not enthusiastic about it they saw that my program was working and did not bar me from taking them.

Keep in mind too that this supplement protocol is an additional expense and you don't have to purchase all of them.

Let's start off with the core supplements which you can find online on Amazon, Vitacost, and health food stores:

- **A Whole Food plant-based multivitamin** without iron (brands I used were Vitacost Synergy, Garden of Life, Deva, Natural Factors, and New Chapter) I took regularly once daily in the morning with my food. Some people may say that if you eat a balanced diet it should be sufficient. What many fail to recognize and understand that a damaged liver and compromised digestive system is not absorbing and assimilating enough vital nutrients to do the massive repair job internally.

- **Vitamin B Complex 100 vitamins** (2x daily with food) for optimal energy production through the conversion of our food into fuel and proper metabolism of proteins, fats, carbohydrates, healthy nervous system. Having a compromised and scarred liver I could feel the difference whenever I missed taking these vitamins. My body was under tremendous stress internally and the B vitamins helped me handle it effectively. The brands I used were Vitacost Synergy, Jarrow, Solgar, VegLife, and GNC depending on what was on sale.

- Vitamin C with Citrus Bioflavonoids 1000 mg. (4x daily with food taken morning, mid-morning, afternoon, and evening) for protection against free radicals, healthy maintenance of my DNA, and improving my body's ability to handle stressors.

- **Natural Vitamin E** with tocotrienols and mixed tocopherols(400 iu 3x daily with food) can reduce the damage that free radicals cause to the body and supports a healthy blood system. Brands I used were Vitacost, Solgar, and Now.

- **Selenium** (200 mcg daily with food) is an important free radical scavenger, maintaining a healthy immune system, health of the thyroid gland, and most important for me was its role in helping my liver function with a number of antioxidant enzyme systems in the body such as glutathione peroxidase. I found best results using the Vitacost Selenium Select and the Vitacost Complexed Selenium-Albion Selenium Glycinate complex.

- **Alpha Lipoic Acid** (600 mg. twice daily with food) or **R-Alpha Lipoic Stabilized Acid** (100 mg twice daily with food). Alpha lipoic acid (ALA and also known as Thioctic Acid) is a natural compound that functions as a co-factor in vital, energy-producing reactions. The body produces very little ALA on its own, and it is difficult to obtain sufficient quantities from diet.

ALA is well known as a powerful antioxidant. It has been called a "universal antioxidant" because it is effective in water-based substances such as blood, while its reduced metabolite, dihydrolipoic acid (DHLA), is effective in fatty tissues and membranes. R-Alpha lipoic acid (RALA) is the naturally occurring form of lipoic acid, a nutrient present in every cell of the body, essential to chemical reactions that allow the body to produce energy. The body produces very little alpha lipoic acid and it is difficult to obtain sufficient quantities through diet alone. The "R" form is considered the biologically active form, identical to that produced by the body. Unlike other forms of lipoic acid, RALA is bioavailable and more stable in the body.

I found this supplement supremely important in managing my type 2 diabetes as it helped shuttle glucose into the cells to be burned off as energy. I started off with Alpha Lipoic Acid and would switch to RALA every three months and alternate between the two forms depending on the sale prices I would find online and in stores in Canada and the United States. It was playing a vital role in helping my liver. It was helping promote cardiovascular health by protecting against free radical damage. It also enhances the antioxidant activity of vitamins C and E and coenzyme Q10.

It may also increase levels of glutathione, the body's most important antioxidant which is produced in the liver.

- **Omega 3 Fatty Acids (1200 mg. EPA & DHA per serving 4x daily with food)** are essential to the body and must be obtained through diet. Fatty fish, like cod, tuna and salmon, are the best sources, but they can also be found in some plant sources and in flaxseed, walnuts and chia seeds. Most people do not eat enough of these foods, however, to obtain optimal amounts of omega-3 nutrients. The Western diet and the processed foods they contain along with the prevalence of the harmful forms of Omega-6 fats in them contribute to the chronic inflammation inside the body. The key word for me from my medical reports were chronic inflammation of my liver and by extension to the rest of my body. I noticed the positive effect these fatty acids had on me. EPA and DHA are well known for their cardioprotective properties, their ability to maintain healthy cognitive function, their potential to support healthy moods and their positive impact on joint comfort and flexibility Higher blood levels of omega-3 essential fatty acids – including EPA and DHA – are associated with a healthier mood and this I can attest to unequivocally.

Make sure your Omega-3 supplements are molecularly distilled especially if using oils from fish to eliminate traces of dioxin, mercury, PCBs and other environmental contaminants. The brands I used were primarily Vitacost Synergy Mega EFA, Carlson Super Omega-3, Nordic Naturals, and Source Naturals.

- **Vitamin D3(at least 5000 iu daily)** plays a myriad role in good health and in my case I found out my levels of this essential vitamin were abnormally low when the autoimmune diagnosis came. My levels were just one-third that of what a normal adult should have. Functions of vitamin D are a wide range from contributing to bone health to supporting a healthy immune system. With my immune system at a dysfunction I had to raise and maintain my daily levels of Vitamin D3.

- Turkey Tail Mushroom(1000 mg 2x daily) also known as Coriolus is one of the best-documented mushrooms in medical research. With a wide spectrum of beneficial properties, Turkey Tail shows much promise in supporting the immune system with its protein-bound and unique polysaccharides. Turkey Tail mushroom mycelium supports beneficial microflora in the digestive and gastrointestinal ecosystem. I learned about this type of mushroom from a naturopathic doctor I was referred to in North Vancouver at that time. He reviewed my nutritional program including all the supplements I was taking and he was impressed that mine was practically complete except for this mushroom. I didn't think twice about adding this to my supplement program and what I noticed was the abdominal discomfort I was experiencing daily disappeared. The brands I used were primarily Host Defense, Planetary Herbals, and Mushroom Wisdom.

- **Probiotics (Multi-strain with at least 50 billion CFU 2x daily on an empty stomach) and Digestive Enzymes (1 with every meal)** work together and helped heal my gut. I didn't have full-blown Irritable Bowel Syndrome (IBS) but I did exhibit symptoms similar to them. Besides, I knew that all the years of continuous antibiotic use when I was younger had shredded my gut and immune system. I didn't realize just how vital a healthy gut was until my bowels started going haywire prior to my hospitalizations. I never want to experience that pain and distress again that is why I take probiotics religiously. I also found that these bacteria helped contribute to a better mood, healthier kidneys and prostate, and I hardly got colds or the flu ever since I started taking them. Nowadays I don't take as high a dose of probiotics as I have transitioned to fermented foods like kombucha, sauerkraut, and kimchi as natural sources. But for this time in my life this was the final piece of the puzzle for me for my nutrition program. When looking for a great multi-strain brand make sure they have Saccharomyces boulardii which supports healthy intestinal epithelium lining integrity, the front line for the body's defense system, plus Lactobacillus and Bifidobacterium probiotics to promote regular bowel function and immune health.

The brands I used were Garden of Life Primal Defense Ultra Probiotics alternated with Vitacost 10-20 Probiotic Formula and for digestive enzymes I have been using Source Naturals Digestive enzymes.

- Milk Thistle(150 mg of standardized to 80% flavonoids as silymarin) is a plant native to the Mediterranean region and indigenous to western and central Europe. It's been used to support health for more than 2,000 years. Milk thistle seeds contain an antioxidant flavonoid complex known as silymarin. This flavonoid helps promote healthy liver function and is also a powerful antioxidant that can help protect healthy cells from free radical damage. The brands I use and trust are Vitacost, Jarrow, Mega Foods, New Chapter, and Now.

Now that you know about the nutrition protocol that helped me heal physically we now turn towards the deeper, more volatile, and topsy-turvy part of it. With my body and brain now being nourished with clean food and drink and providing a boost to my mental focus and clarity I now turned to healing myself on a psychological and emotional level.

The next chapter we will go on a journey deep inside my shadow self, my wounded inner child, to find my light self and start making myself whole, complete and infused with love.

Bear in mind that while all this was happening I kept on exercising and moving my body daily. No matter what I willed myself to do so and I encourage you to dig deep into your own limitless spring of energy. Success is a mindset.

"What we achieve inwardly will change outer reality." —Plutarch

Chapter 7 – I AM Reborn

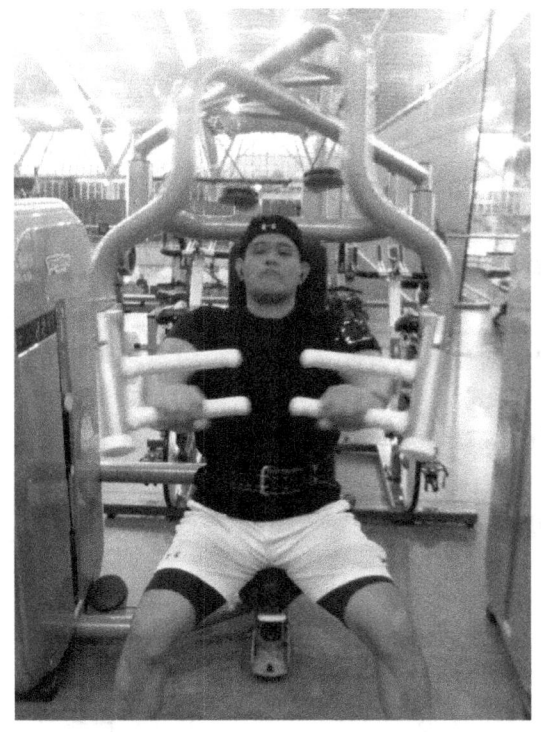

"I am not a product of my circumstances. I am a product of my decisions."

—Stephen Covey

To know what Light truly is you must go into the Darkness and face your greatest fears, your wounded inner child, and do the work necessary so you can accept and love all of You. I realized that this condition that threatened my very life was also my greatest treasure. I had to learn that nothing ever grows in a comfort zone. Creating the nutrition programs necessary for my physical health and recovery was easy compared to the inner work I had to do.

For much of my existence I have lived in a world not my own but rather one that I allowed society, religion, family, and environment to mold and shape me. I once was a child that allowed my emotions, thoughts, and creativity flow with grace and ease. The older I got the more my own personality became submerged through the influence of the desires, actions, and temptations of the false self and I got attached to all its trappings. My life transformed into one of fear and illusions thinking that my liberation, fulfillment, purpose and happiness came from an external magical deity that would grant my wishes and desires as long as I paid homage daily.

This illness and coming face to face with my mortality shattered that glass mirror and started tearing down the walls of doubt and fear. I realized that everything that I aspired for was a lie and that the pursuit of happiness can never be satisfied by material assets and the pleasures and addictions that came with it. I was driven by this toxic and wounded false Masculine energy that had let the

Divine Feminine energy that is a part of me and my other half be submerged in its anger, aggression, greed, jealousy, gluttony, and ignorance. The Feminine energy that flows within each of us and this whole universe that is the nurturing, nourishing, creativity, boundless intuitive wisdom, compassion, kindness, balance and fairness was nearly lost in me.

The amazing aspect of this journey is that this Feminine energy I thought lost was just waiting to be reactivated again. That seed was planted and activated in me when I met Radhaa of Goddess Code Academy and Maya The Shaman of Lemurian Code Healing back in 2011 when I was going through my weight loss transformation and reversing type 2 Diabetes. From 2013 to 2016 I applied all the lessons and knowledge I learned from them to work on myself internally.

I was getting a lot of advice from well-meaning friends and family and I am grateful for their love and support. Love is the ultimate force that helps heal the world and a person. For my deeply wounded body I first had to understand how it got to that point. I shared in my first book how I abused my body with the addictions and pleasures of food and drink. I also shared that through the healing and coaching sessions with Radhaa I was able to heal my unhealthy relationship with food. Radhaa's a master and a conduit at activating the latent Feminine energy codes dormant in each one of us.

The work I needed to do was to go deep inside my wounded self. My liver inflammation and the manifestation of the autoimmune condition was proof that I was peeling away deep layers of negative and toxic energy and belief systems that my real self was rejecting.

She and Maya The Shaman told me back in 2012 that once the healing process begins I would have to go through it and be prepared to do the work. No one else can do the work for one to heal. Now here I was in 2014 allowing my intuition to flow from within. I also had to go inside of me through meditation, journaling, and daily reflection and find that wounded inner child that I had rejected.

I thought that I had healed my wounded self in 2012 when I lost all the weight and reversed type 2 Diabetes. That was just the tip of the iceberg. I had to go back to Vancouver and repair the relationships I had with my family and ultimately myself. I had been away from them and hadn't seen them for over a decade and I was still hiding a lot of pain and emotions from a failed marriage, career, and business. I had a lot of resentment towards the forced worship of a religion I found to be not in alignment anymore with my moral values. There were so many contradictions and I was also disillusioned and angry with myself for allowing the atmosphere of fear swirling around its practice. I was angry with my inner child that got sucked in and became a voiceless sheep to the brainwashing. I was ashamed of my inner child that had so many failures and rejections and insecurities over the years. I was embarrassed for allowing myself to be taken advantage of by unscrupulous individuals throughout my career and in school. I was angry and ashamed that I did not speak up before when I was younger when I wanted to pursue architecture instead of business. I was angry and ashamed that I did not learn how to improve my emotional intelligence and communication with my spouse, my bosses, and friends that took advantage of my kindness and generosity. Most of all I was angry and ashamed of myself for being such a coward and weakling during the times I was expected to step up for myself.

During my meditations this wounded inner child would appear as this crying, whimpering, deeply scarred, scared, horrifically disfigured version of me that hid in the darkness. Initially I recoiled at approaching him. I didn't know what to say and how to say I was so sorry. This kind of internal healing work does not happen in just one sitting. Just as I took the time and took the little steps I made when I was losing weight I had to commit to my inner healing. I had to allow the flow of the Divine Feminine energies to permeate all of me.

While I was doing this inner work I also made a commitment to improve my knowledge of self by reading books and listening to audio books that would uplift me. Between 2013 and 2016 I accumulated a collection of spiritual and motivational books which I kept in my Kindle and my phone for easy access. It didn't matter whether I was at the airport or on the plane, at home in California or back in Vancouver, these books became my wellspring of knowledge. They trained my mind by providing the positive mental nutrition and programming I needed. These books are the following:

- Letting Go: The Pathway of Surrender
- The Surrender Experiment
- A New Earth: Awakening to Your Life's Purpose
- The Seat of The Soul
- The Power Of Intention- Learning to Co-create Your World Your Way

- The Alchemist

- The Four Agreements

- The Gregg Braden Audio Collection

- The Willpower Instinct

- The Hidden Spirituality of Men- Ten Metaphors to Awaken the Sacred Masculine

- Embodying the Divine Masculine of All Truth

- Cultivating The Divine- Healing The Dark Masculine

- I Allowed The Universe to Speak

- Co-Creating at Its Best- A Conversation Between Master Teachers

- The Four Insights- Wisdom, Power, and Grace of the Earthkeepers

- Power Up Your Brain- The Neuroscience of Enlightenment

- Called

- The Mayan Tiles

- Way of The Peaceful Warrior

- The Power of Vulnerability: Teachings of Authenticity, Connection, and Courage

- You're It! On Hiding, Seeking, and Being Found

- The Warrior Within: The Philosophies of Bruce Lee

- The Book of Mastery

- The Light Between Us

- Your Soul's Plan: Discovering the Real Meaning of Life

- The Unlimited Sparks of a Bonfire

- Mindset: The New Psychology of Success

- The Forty Rules of Love: A Novel of Rumi

- Science and The Akashic Field: An Integral Theory of Everything

- Warrior of The Light: A Manual

I didn't know what was guiding me to discover all these resources at that time. It's only now when I was talking to Radhaa and we discussed the Goddess Code Activations™ modality she had created and used on me and her clients when I realized it was the Shakti energy flowing through the different Goddesses that was guiding me all throughout. The Goddess Code Activations™ was the spark that triggered this chain reaction inside of me. I harken back to that night of December 31, 2010 at the beach where I cried out to the universe for salvation. That story in full detail is in my first book and now it had come full circle to this point.

It wasn't just the books and audio books that were coming to me with the flow. I discovered healing meditations I could listen to on YouTube and Soundcloud. I was being led to knowledge, to healing frequencies of light and sound, and I would integrate them into my daily life. Whether I was at the airport, at the gym, the library, the parks, the beaches, and the mountains of Vancouver, Victoria, Los Angeles, and Orange County I found myself being drawn back to nature and reconnecting with the earth and the universe.

I took off my shoes and grounded myself on the sands of the beaches and on the grass at the parks and outside the gym after my workouts. I breathed in with purpose and gratitude and savored the feeling of the air fill my lungs and my body and exhale forcefully the negative energies and toxins inside of me. I envisioned and visualized myself talking to my cells and telling them to heal.

I meditated and found peace and happiness with the use of crystals and stones like amethyst, tourmaline, lapis lazuli, rose quartz, moldovite, selenite, lemurian seed crystals, tiger's eye, hematite, citrine, obsidian, and fluorite. These crystals and stones have healing and protective properties that medical science scoffs at. I didn't care. I was slowly healing myself inside and out and defying the opinions of the outside world. I learned to focus on my chakras and learn of ways to unblock them and let my energy system flow smoothly.

When my parents prayed for me at their apartment and in church I would respect their wishes and do my meditations there too. A thousand rivers lead to the same ocean is a proverb I learned. I cannot reject any part of me anymore. I love and accept all of me and all my life experiences with no exceptions. By owning all of this you take back your power and complete yourself. Does this mean I stay with the religion I was born and raised with? All I can say is that I follow all the paths that lead to the light and back to the Creator.

During my intense workouts at the gym and outdoors I visualized inward that I was healing my damaged cells and regenerating them one by one. Not only was I visualizing my healing I added the power of intention through the emphatic vocal projection by saying to myself, "I am strong! I am healing! I am enough! I am love!" I didn't care who was around me at that time. I was in my own zone and I was determined and committed to see my healing and full recovery. No matter how much pain, how much discomfort and how exhausted I felt I focused on sculpting myself into the true masterpiece I truly am. I would add to this intention by writing affirmations in my journal every night. The most powerful manifestations come after the two words, "I Am" and what you add after that in a powerful and positive fashion will send healing energies back inside your body.

This inner journey and work required me to let go of what no longer served me for my highest good. This also applied to letting go of people in my circle that lowered my vibe and energy. It was crucial to my healing to rid myself of all stressors from food, drink, environment, and people. I discerned and forgave myself and those who had hurt me. I asked for forgiveness from those I had hurt at any time. I learned to step away from situations that placed undue pressure and expectations not beneficial for me. It wasn't about being selfish. You have to practice self-care and self-love on every level for mind, body, and spirit.

There were other physical challenges that came out between 2014 and 2015 which I attributed to a spillover effect from my damaged liver. My hormones got upended and I experienced a severe imbalance that resulted in estrogen dominating my testosterone. My kidney function also was affected along with my prostate. I was diagnosed with sleep apnea. It was later discovered that I had severe food sensitivities triggered by blackberries, blueberries, strawberries, grapefruit, raspberries and sesame seeds that required me to carry an epipen wherever I went just in case. Each new physical challenge that came up I went deeper into myself with my meditations and visualizations. I was being led by the Feminine energies finally activated in me and I responded with love, forgiveness, compassion, and gratitude. I learned to transmute the temporary feelings of anger, sadness, loneliness, and fear through this inner work.

The darkness and shadows wanted to be recognized and accepted and this was the lesson I had to learn. There is no light without darkness and vice versa. The negative energies residing in my cells were not just from my immediate lifetime and lineage. They were from many lifetimes and it was all in that wounded, scared, angry, and lonely inner child that I had rejected before. All of us have that wounded inner child inside of us. We are all imperfect beings on this planet.

In my visualization and meditation exercises I saw my healed, strong and vibrant light form approach that scared, inner child full of scars hiding in the shadows and hug him with love and compassion. As we hugged we began to merge as one and the light began to fill all his scars. The merging completed, I now saw this smiling child with light shining through the scars and he was no longer in pain. We were together now and I would not reject or throw him out ever again. You have to be courageous and face your fears, accept your imperfections and weaknesses, amplify your strengths, harness the nurturing feminine energies that bring balance to the runaway masculine energies.

Practice love, forgiveness, compassion, and gratitude on a daily basis. Do not dwell in pain, shame and anger and allow it to become the reality your earthly self resides in.

It was the Feminine energies that were activated in me by Radhaa's Goddess Code Activations™ and brought me to this miraculous self-healing to continue the work of shining love and light to this world that needs it. My work is just beginning.

This healing was validated in this reality in 2016 by my doctor here in California through the blood tests they ran. My doctor just shook his head as he looked at my medical records and told me that it looked like I had never gotten sick. Believe in miracles because in you is the answer to everything. You are the Light and the Love you have always been.

"Everything you've ever wanted is on the other side of fear."—George Addair

Chapter 8 – I AM Light and Love

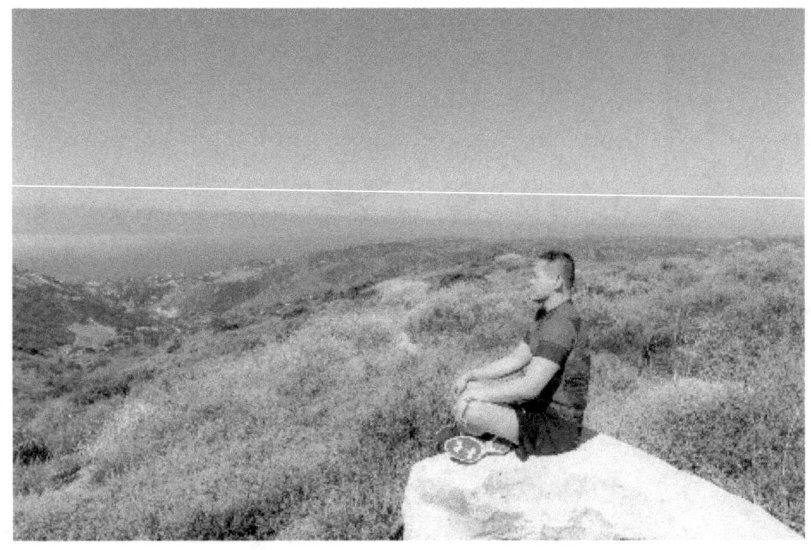

We are all just visitors to this time, this place, this reality. We are all just passing through so let's enjoy the view and the Now. We are here to observe, to learn, to grow, to evolve, and to love. Then when it's time...we return Home. Let yourself evolve into your true purpose.

Where is home? It's not a magical place that's outside of us. It's inside of us and all around us. It's everywhere and everything. We are all a part of this Universe. What did this illness teach me? It taught me to find my true self by reconnecting the Divine Feminine and Sacred Masculine and shine a beacon of light and love to inspire those who feel they are trapped in the darkness.

My daily life is one where I start with gratitude for a new day given as a gift. To be aware that there is abundance, prosperity and blessings everywhere. Before I partake of any food and drink I say this:

"Thank you for this food and drink I am about to partake. Thank you to those who through their love, work, and diligence brought this blessing to me. It heals me, nourishes me, strengthens me, and energizes me."

From my spiritual coaches Radhaa and Maya The Shaman I also learned to say daily Baba Nam Kevalam which means, "Love is all there is."

The following passages I highly encourage you to read out loud for yourself with passion and conviction. Let the power of intention

I honor and love my body through exercise and movement. I acknowledge, accept and commit that by this exercise and movement that it produces healing energy that rejuvenates, strengthens, and inspires me. This illness does not define me or hinder me. It is a part of me that I love and fully accept as a treasure.

I honor and love my mind through enriching it with positivity, reading, meditating, singing, laughing, encouraging creativity and feeding it daily with beautiful intentions, stimulating it by writing out those intentions as affirmations and taking action with ease and grace.

I honor and love my spirit by letting my light shine through and letting love be the ultimate force that radiates from it. I am Light and I am Love.

I honor and love my family, my friends and all of humanity by respecting them, listening to them, understanding them, empathizing with them, practicing kindness daily, setting boundaries that respects myself and them, and not taking anything personally.

I honor and love all of myself and acknowledge, love and accept that my existence represents the eternal union within and without between the Divine Feminine and Divine Masculine.

Enjoy life in the present. Be grateful for the lessons and experiences of the past. Live life fully and go for your dreams. Don't be attached to external material stuff that doesn't matter. Prioritize and treasure memories instead of things. The past has already happened. Learn from it. It is a part of who you are. Don't worry about the future for it hasn't happened yet. Focus on the present and making today the best and happiest day ever.

Spend time with yourself and the ones you love. Let them know you love them by telling them. Spread love, joy, positivity, gratitude, and happiness instead of hate, blame, and negativity.

Take care of yourself and love yourself. Look in the mirror and smile. You are beautiful. You are strong. You are limitless. Forgive yourself and others. By doing this it liberates you from its heaviness and attracts more abundance and blessings your way.

Change is uncomfortable but necessary for growth. Don't be a servant to your mind. Once you condition your mind to accept that change is good then it becomes a habit that it just does. The true path to liberation lies in your ability to not be attached to the desires and temptations of this material world.

Let the Dvine Feminine energies activate and seep into your life and let it be your strength just as it did mine. Let the true Divine Masculine awaken and say enough to the asshole model of this patriarchal, ego-based controlling energy. Through this illness I saw that this was the corrupt, flawed and dangerous energy that almost killed me. A true aspect of the Divine Masculine is strength. Not in the perverted form we see acted out today. It's a strength that comes from inside, from spirit. This is found in both men and women.

Connected to strength because of the feminine energies that allowed me to go inward and then outward with my masculine aspect. It's about fighting the good fight and not fighting others. I am a warrior that fights for the truth. This illness revealed the truth not just for myself but for everyone else. I learned about power and about setting up clearly defined boundaries so that no one would ever walk through me again. It didn't matter if it was family or friend. I would never attack another but if you attack me and try to abuse me I will fight back and defend myself and prevent you from doing that.

It doesn't matter what obstacles you face. The Divine Masculine helps overcome all. What I learned too about the power of the Divine Masculine is that it comes from knowing who you truly are. It wasn't obtained through tricks and shortcuts nor was it taken from someone else. Along with that the other aspects and traits of the Divine Masculine are determination, resilience and focus.

I knew where I wanted to go, visualized it beforehand and savored the feeling of being healed and full of strength and energy, and I refused to let go of that dream. Then I went out and created the foundation. Guided by the Divine Feminine Goddess energies that flowed through me I found the materials to build with to heal my body and then integrated it with the mental and spiritual exercises I have outlined here. You too can do this to heal yourself and overcome any obstacles. Let the Divine Feminine and Divine Masculine come together and activate in you. Be open to all the possibilities and step out of that box you were put in by the world. What happens next is magical and beautiful.

"Too many of us are not living our dreams because we are living our fears." —Les Brown

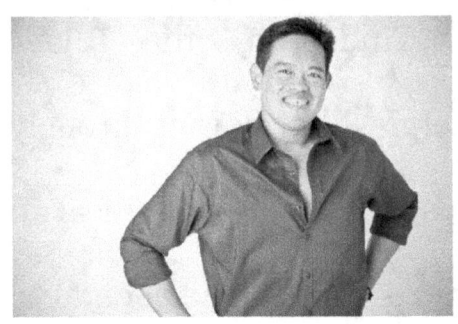

ABOUT THE AUTHOR

Michael Pestano is a business, health and wellness coach, a certified fitness trainer specializing in sports nutrition and weight loss, and a motivational speaker . He is devoted to complete holistic wellness and a preventive approach to illness. He is the oldest of four children and was born and raised in the Philippines before migrating with his family to Canada. After living there for fourteen years he moved to the United States. He has been in the natural health industry since 1998 and dedicated to share to the world the benefits of living a healthy lifestyle in mind, body, and spirit.

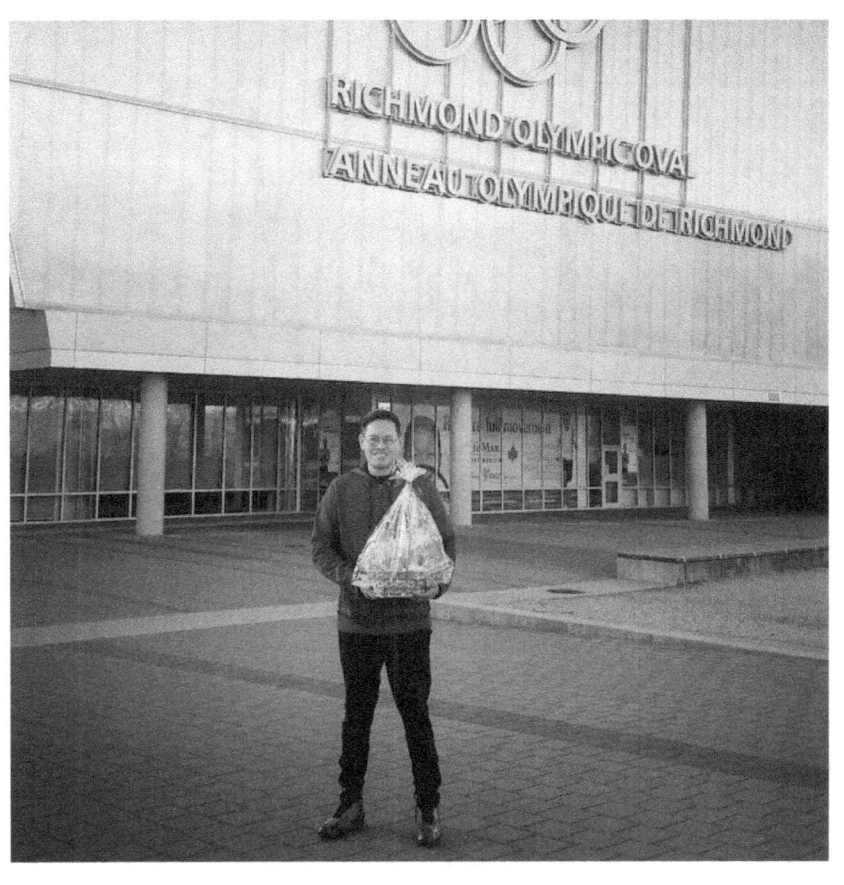

2015 Richmond Olympic Oval Winner

Member Challenge